D0486191

HAND REFLEXOLOGY: KEY TO PERFECT HEALTH

Mildred Carter

Parker Publishing Company, Inc.

West Nyack, New York

© 1975 *by*

Parker Publishing Company, Inc.
West Nyack, New York

Reward Edition . . . . . June 1977

Library of Congress Cataloging in Publication Data

Carter, Mildred.
    Hand reflexology--key to perfect health.

    1. Reflexotherapy. I. Title. [DNLM: 1. Hand--
Popular works. 2. Massage--Popular work. 3. Reflexo-
therapy--Popular works. WB960 C324h]
RM723.C5C34   615'.822   74-26152

Printed in the United States of America

To my son, Kenneth Nelson; to my two daughters, Verlee Paul and Tammy Weber; and to my husband, Noah Frank Powell. Also, to all who are searching for a natural way to health, that they may find in Reflexology a path to a happier, healthier future for themselves and their families.

ACKNOWLEDGMENTS

My special thanks go to Dr. Lloyd B. Rapp, N.D., Sutherlin, Oregon, Dr. H. A. Hagan, D.C., Cottage Grove, Oregon and Dr. J. P. Schaller, D.C., of Paradise, California, for their counsel and help; and to Dr. R. C. Wilborn, D.C., N.D., of Health Research, Mokelumne Hill, California, for giving me permission to use material from several of his books.

Also, thanks to the many chiropractors for their cooperation and help in compiling this book; and to Dr. James Brandt for his part in making it possible for me to continue my research into this ancient healing art of Reflexology.

I am also indebted to Stirling Enterprises, Inc., Cottage Grove, Oregon, for their cooperation in supplying materials for demonstration in photographs; and to Jack Hausotter, Roseburg, Oregon, for his help in supplying some of the illustrations for this book.

Especially do I want to thank Mrs. Hilda E. Peterson for her valuable and skilled editorial help and enthusiastic support in launching this book; also Verlee Paul and Tammy Weber for help in obtaining models and special photographs; and to Pat Fitting for her individual help in typing, and my very dear friend, Jessie L. Baker, for always being available when needed. Also, to the National Health Federation, Monrovia, California, for the helpful information derived from their monthly bulletins.

And most of all, I wish to thank my husband, Noah Frank Powell, for his help, understanding, and patience over a period of two years during which the preparation of this book took most of my time.

Foreword

It gives me much pleasure to add a few lines to Mildred Carter's fascinating book on reflex-massage. My attention to this field and its therapeutic value was drawn by my learned friend Aslam Effendi, who, among other things, is a student of the Carter school and has been giving convincing demonstrations of the techniques outlined in this book for laymen. For example, abnormal conditions in the body show up in the hands and feet; and no such reflexes are found in healthy people.

Many centuries back, the Chinese physicians discovered acupuncture, and something similar was practiced in the Indo-Pakistan sub-continuent. But it was only in the beginning of this century that some medical pioneers in the West improved on the techniques of the ancient oriental physicians by developing Reflexology (or western-type acupuncture). And, today, Reflexology can certainly prove an effective weapon in the hands of physiotherapists and the medical profession generally. Perhaps it was the pioneering work of Reflexologists that inspired Elizabeth Kenny to develop her technique to combat poliomyelitis, and thus gain world recognition despite bitter opposition from the medical profession.

As a physician and scientist, I have learnt one very important lesson—and that is to be always a humble and curious student. Therefore, Mildred Carter, and pioneers like her, who are trying in their own humble way to unveil some of the vast mysteries of the healing art, deserve our respectful attention.

Z. Hussain,
M.B., B.S.
Consulting Physician
Pakistan

Preface

This book is written in response to many requests from people who were introduced to the wonderful healing powers of reflex massage as described in my former book, "Helping Yourself With Foot Reflexology," and who find it difficult to use the techniques on their feet for various reasons. Since "hand massage" is mentioned in the book, they have requested detailed information on reflexes in the hands.

The hands contain the same reflexes as the feet, but in different locations and require their own rules for locating these "miracle buttons" which bring prompt relief from many ailments as well as renewed health and vitality to every part of the body through simple but effective manipulation.

For those who have not read my former book, it will be necessary to repeat some of the information given in order that a book limited to hand massage may be as complete as possible in itself.

Hand reflexology is so simple that it can be used anywhere by anyone—hunters, athletes, students, sportsmen, executives, and housewives. It can be used indoors or out in any occupation or activity, with perfect safety, by following a few simple rules.

The reader is cautioned, however, that there are some conditions which may require the attention of a medical doctor or chiropractor, and when this is the case, common sense dictates that such care should be sought.

M.C.

Brief History
of Reflexology

Although the principles of reflex massage have been known for centuries, with the advance of medical science it was slowly discarded for newer innovations, not always any better and requiring considerable experimentation not only with animals, but also with humans.

Reflexology was re-discovered by Dr. William Fitzgerald in 1913 and brought to the attention of the medical world. To quote from "Health Counselor," he states "Zone therapy (as it was called) has been practiced and taught by some of the most noted doctors in America."

Doctor Joe Selby Riley (M.D., M.S., D.O., N.D.) said, "The scope of the science of Zone Reflex (reflexology) is almost unlimited. Great physicians who have investigated it fully made the claim that it is the greatest ally yet found to their work. Side by side with other great therapies, zone therapy will stand in the march of science and progress."

Reflexology has been retained in health centers by professional reflexologists, but the general public has been so exposed to pills, salves, ointments, tranquilizers, and surgery of an offending organ, that the man on the street looks with askance at the principle of massaging a reflex in the hands or feet to treat an ailing organ far distant in the body.

Reflexology is one of the most miraculous means of utilizing nature's own healing methods for maintaining the body in peak operating condition, and probably one of the least familiar to us. It requires no pills, drugs, tranquilizers, or mutilating surgery, can be self-administered with perfect safety, anywhere or anytime, and can be used with people of all ages.

The body's vital life force circulates along pathways, and we can tap it at an estimated 800 points on the body. It is not necessary to know all of these points since the hands as well as the feet contain "reflex buttons" which are connected to all organs and glands, and when these reflex centers are massaged, they send a stimulating surge of new vigor to whatever part of the body they are connected to, instantly and with no after-effects such as we often suffer from medications. We are correcting imbalance in this primary flow and thereby helping nature do the healing.

This book shows how you can use this "push button" method of massage with illustrations, charts, and easy-to-follow massage techniques.

I constantly search for new methods of natural healing, and when I find one that is better than the positive and simple methods of reflexology, I will bring this method to you.

You need no longer live in fear of so-called incurable diseases: *nothing is incurable*:—diseases are the result of malfunctioning of the cells and imperfection of the body tissues due to unnatural elements of living. Just turn to nature and give her a chance to put your body chemistry back into normal performance by rebuilding perfect cells and new healthy tissues for your whole body.

How This Book
Came to Be Written

It seems that I was born with a desire to help the sick and injured. As long as I can remember, I was rescuing and doctoring animals and birds and even bugs.

When I was very young, I remember rescuing prairie dogs that my father had gassed or poisoned. They were a great nuisance on the ranches, and the farmers were trying to exterminate them. I was gathering all the sick ones and doctoring them back to health until my father found my "clinic."

When I was about seven, I experienced a cure of the general weakness I had suffered from since early babyhood. No one knew what it was. When we moved to California, I met some children eating garlic. I couldn't seem to get enough of it. My poor mother was an understanding person and let me eat all I wanted even though she couldn't stand me near her because of the strong garlic odor. I was never sick again after that "garlic binge." I have since studied the wonderful healing powers of garlic and herbs. I think this experience has always stayed with me and slanted my interest toward other natural systems of cures for various illnesses.

When my husband was stricken with a heart attack in his early 30's, no doctor knew what to do for him. They knew very little about heart disease at that time. So I turned to prayer, studied diet where I could, and he had a very quick recovery. That is when I wrote my first book, *The Power of Thought.* When my husband passed away eight years later from virus pneumonia, the doctors said that by all the laws of nature he should never have lived through the heart attack he had suffered years earlier.

I thought of studying to be a medical doctor but decided against it. If I did that, I would know only what doctors know. So I devoted my life to studying all phases of natural healing, of which there are many. But, to date, I have not found any method of physical healing which equals the simple, natural, and safe way to health that *reflexology* offers—a method of healing that anyone can use on himself or his family in complete safety with the most remarkable results.

AMAZING QUICK RECOVERIES

In my years of practicing reflexology, I have never gotten over being amazed at the quick relief people received from so many ailments. It was as if I pushed a magic button to instant health, in many cases. They would come into the office doubled up with pain and completely hopeless, convinced that such a simple thing as massaging and pressing certain points in the feet and hands could not possibly help, but their mother or a neighbor had insisted that they come. Then the amazed look on their faces when the pain actually stopped, sometimes in seconds!

REFLEXOLOGY SEEMS LIKE A MIRACLE

It gave me great satisfaction to watch people recuperate under my very eyes in just a short time, some taking longer than others, of course. Mr. A. came to me for treatments for over five years, not because he had anything the matter with him after the first few treatments, but because he liked the feeling of vitality and well-being that he felt after each treatment. He brought his mother from a great distance on many occasions, just to make sure she remained in good health.

These reflexology treatments are in no way miraculous, although they may seem that way. They merely open the channels so that the normal healing process can be speeded up by supplying more energy to the right places and thus aid nature in her work of repairing your body.

A good, full flow of water cannot run through a clogged or rusty pipe—the pipe must be cleaned of all obstructions to get the full flow of water through. This is true of your veins, the nerves, and also the network of invisible channels.

TESTIMONIALS PROVE REFLEXOLOGY WORKS

I can give you not hundreds, but thousands, of case histories I receive through the mail from people all over the world telling me of the wonderful results they are getting by using the simple method of reflex massage. The following unsolicited testimonials are typical samples.

Unity Ministers Call Reflexology Magic

Mrs. M. and I feel that you are our friend through your rich sharing with us in the book on Foot Reflexology, West Nyack, N.Y.: Parker Publishing Company, Inc., 1969.)

In the middle thirties we were ministers in Unity in Rochester, N.Y. The president of the board was Mr. G. About twenty years later I returned to Rochester for a visit, and while in the home of Mr. and Mrs. G., they told us of a new magic in healing which they had heard about and tested and were made believers, and it was all about a technique of working on the feet.

We forgot about the incident until recently we learned about your book and ordered it. I have been reading and studying it diligently (my wife says she thinks I am reading it more than the Bible).

May God continue to bless you in your continued ministry of healing.

Sincerely and gratefully,
Rev. L.M.

How Reflexology Changed My Life

Your book, "Helping Yourself with Foot Reflexology," has changed my life. Would you believe that I cured myself of life-long headaches within *three minutes* by following your directions? And as an added bonus I cured myself of chronic canker sores at the very same time. I mean to tell you that canker sores healed up at once, immediately, the very same time as my headaches were cured.

The very first night I slept completely through the night, never getting up once to go to the bathroom. All this happened to me the very first day. Unbelievable but true. Thanks to you.

You will be happy to learn that two of our friends were

cured of hemorrhoids within *three weeks*. Two of our friends living here were cured of prostate trouble within *three days*. They followed the directions in your book.

We are so indebted to you, Mrs. Carter, and the only way I can repay you is to tell all of our friends and relatives of your wonderful book.

Thank you and kindest regards.

Sincerely and gratefully yours,
J.P., California

A Doctor Chiropodist-Podiatrist Has Success with Reflex Massage

I am getting some good results with a few patients and friends of mine. Would like to know if there is anyone doing the work in this area. I have people I could refer to them for treatments.

I find the book very interesting and helpful.

Sincererly,
A.D.D., D.S.C.

You can see why I want to give everyone the natural healing methods of reflexology by these simple methods of pressing reflex buttons on your hands, or your feet. You may find one system more effective than the other.

You can activate a vital life force into all parts of your body (or of someone else if you wish) for renewed magnetic energy for a fuller, happier, healthful life.

The Author

CONTENTS

1

What This Book
Will Do for You

There is a healing energy which circulates through the body on specific pathways, which were mapped out centuries ago by man. This energy we call "life force" or "vital energy." Although this force can be "tapped" at more than 800 points, this book shows you how to tap this healing current to bring natural and prompt relief from practically all your aches and pains, chronic or acute, by the simple process of massaging the "reflex buttons" located in your hands, which are connected to all your glands, organs, and the nervous system.

The techniques of reflex massage are fully illustrated by diagrams and photographs in simple self-help steps showing how the various reflexes "signal" the presence of a malfunction in some gland or organ in the body and how to send a surge of healing energy for prompt relief of the condition, merely by pressing and massaging the reflex connected to it. This method of restoring the body to normal functioning involves no expense, no special equipment, no drugs or medication. The results are amazingly fast, bringing relief often in a matter of *seconds*.

A glance at the Table of Contents will indicate the wide range of situations for which reflexology has been used to obtain beneficial results. Reflex massage can not only cure specific ailments but can be used to keep you in good health and build resistance to attacks of disease. In addition, the method detects health problems before they become serious. You will gain more youthful energy, and learn

21

how to reduce health-destroying mental and physical tensions.

The simple technique of reflex massage can be used and applied at any time and practically anywhere. For instance, if you are suffering from a headache while attending a meeting, you can quickly stop the pain without anyone being the wiser. Or, you can take a "reflex break" for a fast pickup of energy—in your office, while visiting, and even while driving the car.

The book also contains case histories which the author has experienced in her years of practice in the healing art of reflexology, as well as from medical doctors who have recognized the natural healing properties of reflex massage using various techniques for stimulating the reflexes. In addition, there are letters the author has received from all over the world telling of personal experiences and recovery from illnesses through reflexology.

Reflexology is nature's "push button" secret for dynamic living, abundant physical energy, vibrant health, better living without pain, retaining youthful vigor, and enjoying life to the fullest as is man's birthright, and by keeping this book within easy reach for reference when confronted with a health problem, you can get all these benefits and even more.

THE ANCIENT MEDICAL BOOKS EXPLAIN

A basic philosophy was explained in ancient medical books that health is dependent upon the balance and maintenance of harmony within the body.

To obtain this balance there must be a free and unimpeded circulation of energy flowing through the body's organs.

The aim of reflexology is to break down the blockage and restore the free flow of energy or life force through these invisible channels.

There are more than 800 pressure points that the Chinese use. Some chiropractors are familiar with many of these pressure points in the body and use them without the patients being aware of what they are doing. Many are now using foot reflexology to some extent with very gratifying results.

REFLEXOLOGY USED IN MANY COUNTRIES

In studying the relation between acupuncture, not only of the

Chinese, but from its use in other countries as well, we learn that the traditional medicine is based on the belief that the blood circulation follows the flow of energy. This energy circulates freely in an endless cycle from the main organs through the channels beneath the skin. If it is blocked at some point, the circulation is impaired. This blockage results in a deficient oxygenation of the tissues around the affected area and throws the body off balance. This imbalance produces malfunctioning not only of the tissues surrounding it, but, if not corrected, spreads to related organs near by.

Naturalogists show that civilized man's environment and habits make his blood either the sparkling river of life or the stagnant stream of death.

As the toxins of the cells accumulate in the blood, due to man's environment and faulty habits, the body becomes flooded, shocked, and poisoned by its own excrement.

HOW YOU GET INSTANT RELIEF WITH REFLEXOLOGY

Thus you can readily see why you get instant relief when you massage certain points in the hands or the feet. You are loosening the crystals or blockage of these channels which were impairing circulation, thus allowing a free flow of the energy life force to resume its natural flow through the channels so that the body swings back into a natural balance, and harmony and health are once again established. It is so simple when one knows how it works. It is like running fresh water into a muddy, stagnant pool. As soon as there is a continuous supply of clear water, the pool becomes sparkling and clear, full of life and beauty. We don't have to go far to see dead bodies of water in this day. Would that it could be as simple to start a fresh supply of water to them as it is for you to start your spring of life forces circulating in your body for renewal of sparkling health!

ARE YOU CONFUSED?

Are you confused about your health? The more books you read, the more lectures you hear, the more confused you become. Every book and every lecturer, and every authority on health gives you a different answer, often contradictory. They will all point out their different special roads to glorious health.

Optimum health and freedom from disease start with correct and reliable information—information that has been proved by many, by people like you, people who have proved its worth by putting it to use; information from doctors who have proved it enough to use it in their practice.

I am giving you information that will tell you how you can use this art of natural healing that will prevent premature aging and help you to live longer in good health and freedom from disease.

Reflexology Not Confusing

Reflexology is not confusing nor is it contradictory in any form. In this simple, easy to use, harmless, yet scientific, way to health, you can learn how to stop pain all over your body in a matter of seconds in many cases.

Even though your situation is precarious and at times seems hopeless, your self-preservation instinct tells you not to give up. You have become disillusioned by the promises of the great progress of technological, chemical, medical, and pharmacological science to improve the quality of life by eliminating diseases and providing you with an easier and happier life. These promises will never materialize as long as there is greed in man. In 1971, there were an estimated 71 billion dollars paid out on illnesses, and the figure increases with the years.

People who are turning back to nature are experiencing the joys of regained health with little or no expense involved. *Natural health is free.*

2

Guide to Reflexology
Hand Charts

Let us study briefly the reflexology charts of the hands as they follow below for a moment, to get acquainted with the positions of the reflexes in the hands and their corresponding relation to the vital parts of the body. All diagrams in the hands represent *Reflex Areas*.

I have purposely made the diagrams of the organs and glands, etc. small in order to place them all in the small area allowed in the hand, to make it easier for you to identify them.

Explanation of Zone Chart #1

Chart #1 shows ten vertical lines running down through the body. These lines are numbered from 1 through 5 on each side of the body, starting from the tips of the fingers and ending at the tips of the toes. These meridian lines are clues to help you locate the reflexes to certain areas in the body. You will be referring to this chart often as you study the forthcoming chapters.

Explanation of Chart #2

Look closely at Chart #2. Notice how the right hand corresponds to the right side of the body and the left hand to the left side of the body. If you get a clear picture of this in your mind, then it will be simpler for you to find the reflexes in your hands when you are learning to massage them.

I have purposely placed the position of the hands in this chart as

ZONE THERAPY

CHART No. 1

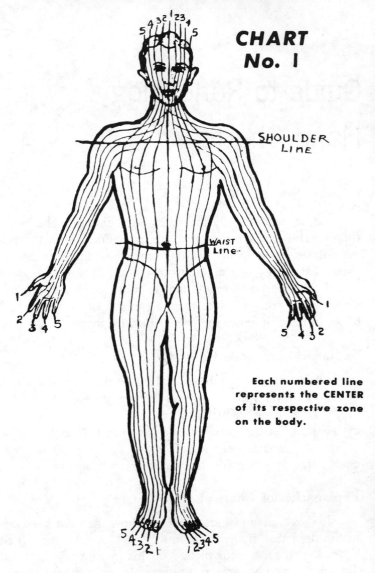

SHOULDER LINE

WAIST Line

Each numbered line represents the CENTER of its respective zone on the body.

Chart #1

26

REFLEX HAND CHART-2

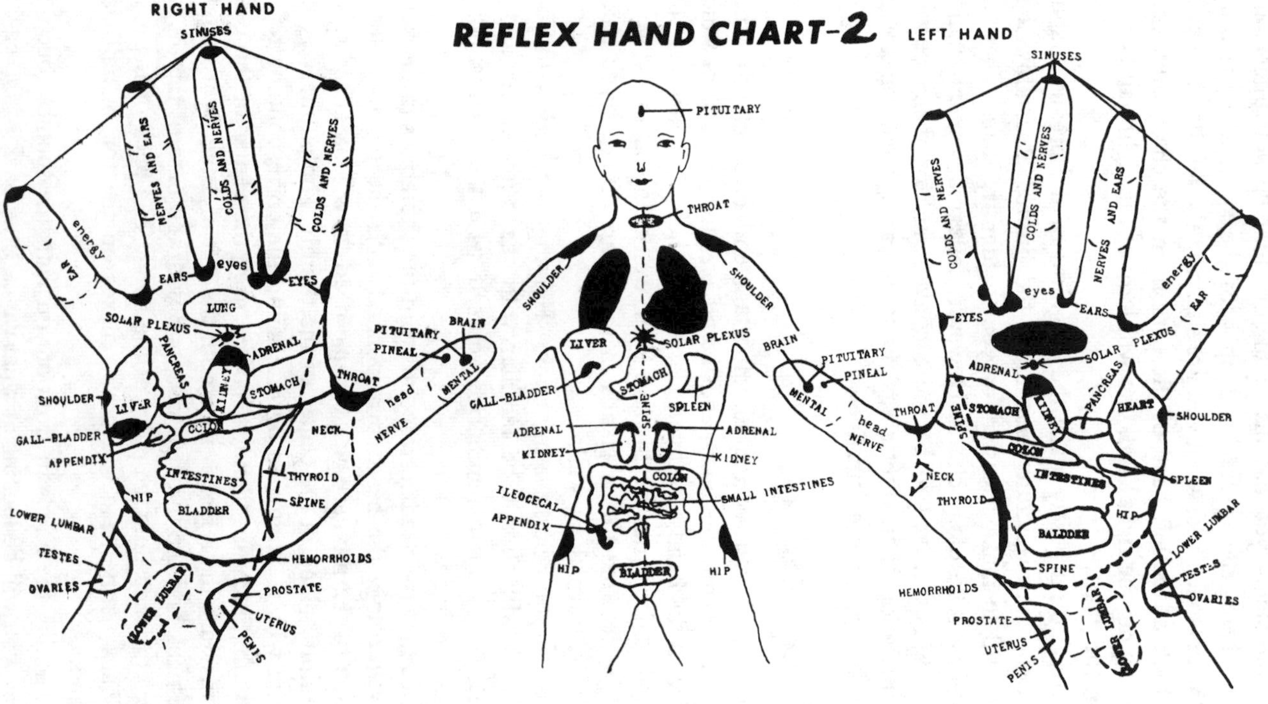

RIGHT HAND

LEFT HAND

Chart #2

SINUSES
COLDS AND NERVES
EYES
COLDS AND NERVES
eyes
EARS
NERVES AND EARS
ENERGY
EAR
SHOULDER
GALL-BLADDER
SOLAR PLEXUS
PANCREAS
LUNG
ADRENAL
LIVER
KIDNEY
STOMACH
COLON
INTESTINES
APPENDIX
HIP
BLADDER
LOWER LUMBAR
TESTES
OVARIES
PITUITARY
PINEAL
MENTAL
BRAIN
head
THROAT
NERVE
NECK
THYROID
SPINE
HEMORRHOIDS
PROSTATE
UTERUS
PENIS
LOWER LUMBAR

PITUITARY
THROAT
SHOULDER
SOLAR PLEXUS
SPINE
LIVER
GALL-BLADDER
ADRENAL
KIDNEY
SPLEEN
ADRENAL
KIDNEY
COLON
ILEOCECAL
APPENDIX
SMALL INTESTINES
HIP
HIP
BLADDER
BRAIN

SINUSES
COLDS AND NERVES
EYES
COLDS AND NERVES
eyes
EARS
NERVES AND EARS
ENERGY
EAR
SHOULDER
HEART
PANCREAS
SPLEEN
SOLAR PLEXUS
ADRENAL
KIDNEY
STOMACH
SPINE
COLON
INTESTINES
BLADDER
HIP
SPINE
LOWER LUMBAR
LOWER LUMBAR
TESTES
OVARIES
PENIS
UTERUS
PROSTATE
HEMORRHOIDS
THYROID
NECK
head
THROAT
NERVE
MENTAL
PINEAL
PITUITARY
BRAIN

27

if the person facing you has his palms up, to help you understand better how these reflexes are lined up with the spine and the other parts of the person. Thus, when you are studying the left hand reflexes, you will look at the left hand of the person on the chart, and when you are studying the right hand, you will look at the right hand of the person on the chart.

I have also purposely made the diagrams of the .organs, glands, etc. small enough to picture them all in the limited area allowed in the hand, and to make it easier for you to identify them. They are similar to foot reflexology charts. However, reflexology manipulation of the hands has proved to be more convenient, for many people, than manipulation of the foot areas. In some cases, hand reflexology proved to be even more effective.

Explanation of Chart #3

In Chart #3 you see the all important endocrine glands which secrete hormones into the body, and the reflexes to these glands which are located in the hands. You will learn in forthcoming chapters how these glands affect your health and your well-being in many ways. You will be referred to the glands in this chart often as you study this book, so learn them well.

Those of you who have my book, "Helping Yourself With Foot Reflexology," will already be familiar with the body charts and it will be easy for you to familiarize yourself with the corresponding reflexes in the hands.

Notice how the head corresponds with the thumb, as in the book on foot reflexology the head corresponded with the big toe. Notice the position of the pituitary gland in the head, now look at the reflex to the pituitary gland in the center of the thumb. The pituitary gland in the head will be stimulated by massaging the corresponding reflex in the thumb. Since this gland is located near the center of the head you will massage the reflex to it in both the left and the right thumb.

The neck and the throat correspond with the base of the thumb where it is fastened onto the palm of the hand. The back of the neck and the back of the head will have reflexes on the top or nail side of the hand.

By holding the hands in front of you with the thumbs touching each other, you will be looking at what we call the back of the hands. If you turn them over with the little fingers touching each other, you will be looking at the palm. In your charts you will be looking at the palms, as this is where we do most of our massaging to send

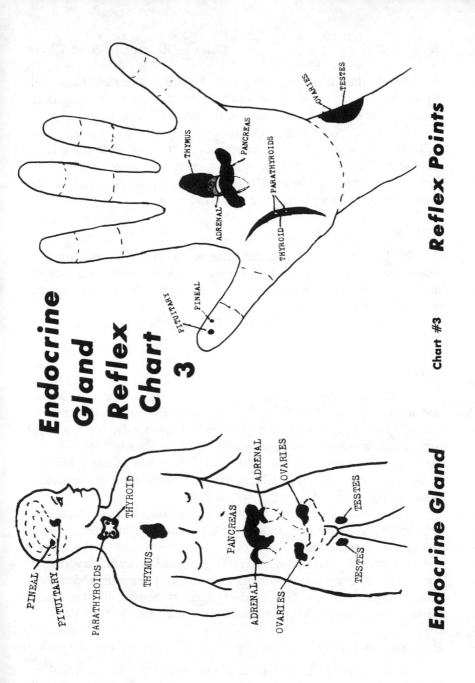

Endocrine Gland Reflex Chart 3

Reflex Points

THYMUS

PANCREAS

ADRENAL

PARATHYROIDS

THYROID

OVARIES

TESTES

PITUITARY

PINEAL

Chart #3

PINEAL

PITUITARY

PARATHYROIDS

THYROID

THYMUS

PANCREAS

ADRENAL

ADRENAL

OVARIES

OVARIES

TESTES

TESTES

Endocrine Gland

currents of vital life force surging into the body, stimulating any and all malfunctioning areas of the body, from the tips of the fingers to the tips of the toes, as explained in the Zone Chart #1.

If you hold your hands up with your fingers close together, you will see that there is about as much area in the fingers as there is in the palm of the hand. This is why so many of the reflexes can be contacted in the fingers as well as the hands, especially when we are anesthetizing in specific cases of localized pain.

Eye and Ear Reflexes

Notice that the eye and ear reflexes on your chart #2 are just below the fingers; since we have an eye and an ear on each side of the head, there will be reflexes on each hand. The reflexes to the right eye and ear will be found on the fingers of the right hand, and the reflexes to the left eye and ear will be found on the fingers of the left hand.

Various Other Reflexes

Notice how the reflex to the liver is located on the right hand, and the liver in the body is on the right side. The heart is on the left side of the body; on the chart you see the reflex to the heart in a corresponding area on the left hand.

The appendix is on the right side of the body at the beginning of the colon, under the liver; the corresponding reflex to the appendix is on the right hand, below the liver reflex.

You should now be getting an idea of how the position of the reflexes in the hands corresponds to the location of the organs and the glands in the body.

By studying this chart you will get a fuller understanding of your body and the corresponding reflexes in your hands. Study it until you have the location of the organs somewhat fixed in your mind, in accordance with the reflex to each one.

Summary of Charts

After studying the charts and the following photos, you can understand how pressing and massaging the reflexes in your hands will stimulate the whole body. You will not be treating just one congested area. You will be sending a flow of the energetic universal forces that created you charging throughout your entire system, in addition to dealing with a specific health situation.

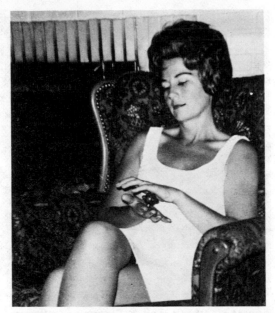

Figure 1. Getting into position to massage reflexes in both hands with the Magic Reflex Massager.

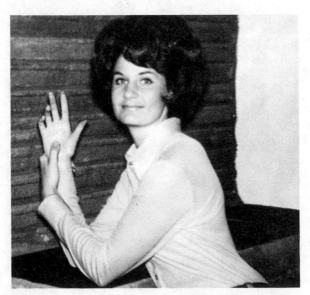

Figure 2. Shows thumb pressing into the reflexes to the colon and the intestines.

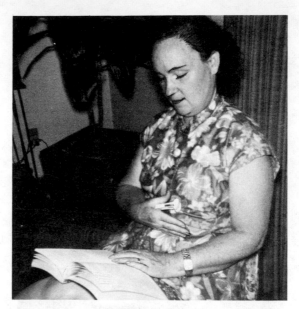

Figure 3. Using Reflex Clamp on reflexes in web of right hand to stimulate the liver.

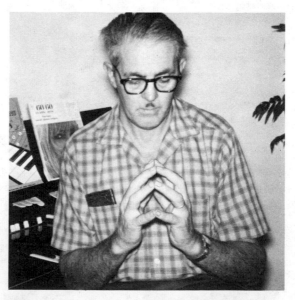

Figure 4. Relieving tension by pressing tips of fingers together.

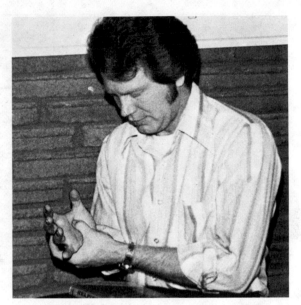

Figure 5. Position for massaging reflexes to the thyroid gland.

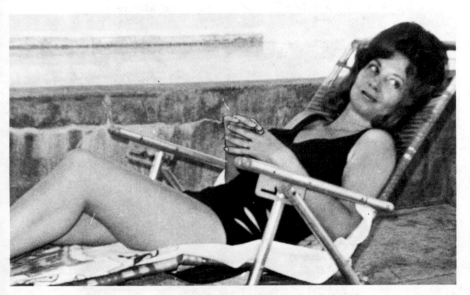

Figure 6. Massaging the reflexes in the web between fingers to relieve headache and tension.

33

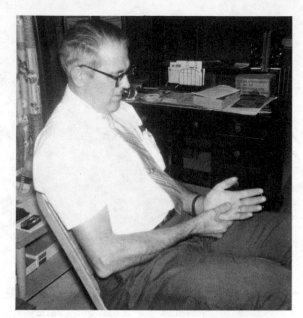

Figure 7. Business executive massaging reflexes to the heart from little finger to center of hand; also the adrenals and kidneys.

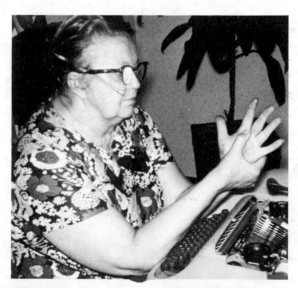

Figure 8. Massaging reflexes to relax eye tension and relieve headache during coffee break.

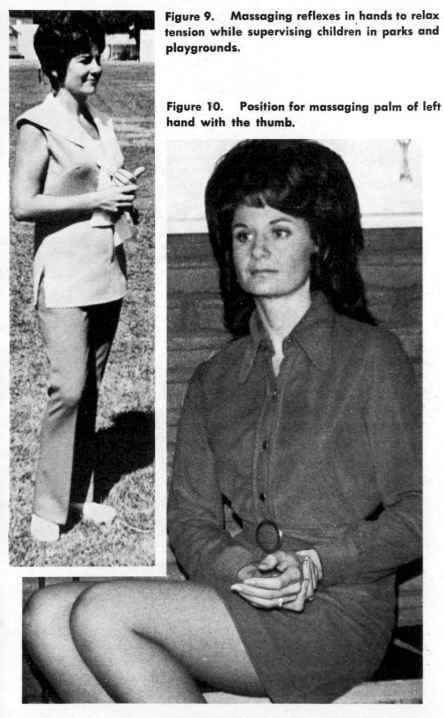

Figure 9. Massaging reflexes in hands to relax tension while supervising children in parks and playgrounds.

Figure 10. Position for massaging palm of left hand with the thumb.

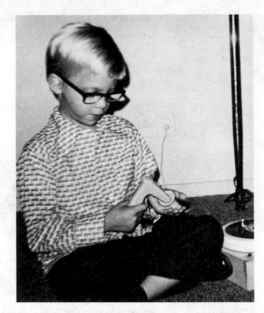

Figure 11. Shows the simplicity of using the Rollo Massager.

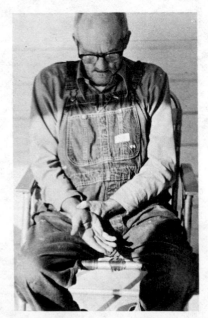

Figure 12. Grandpa massaging reflexes to prostate gland.

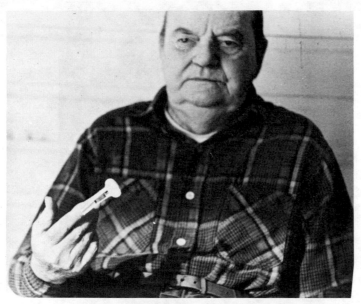

Figure 13. Shows Reflex Clamp on finger #2 for right eye and areas along meridian line 2.

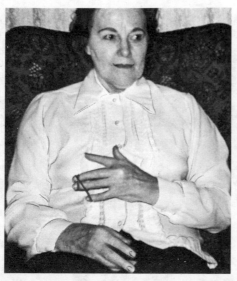

Figure 14. Using rubber bands to relieve pain on left side of head and body. Zones 3, 4, and 5.

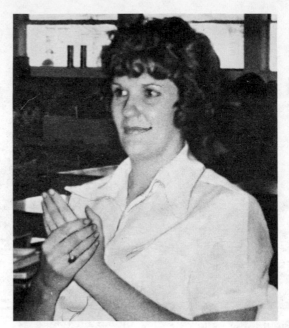

Figure 15. Massaging hands to relieve nervous tension in school room.

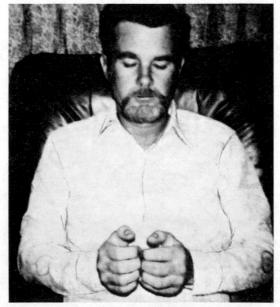

Figure 16. Position for buffing fingernails to stimulate the regrowth of hair.

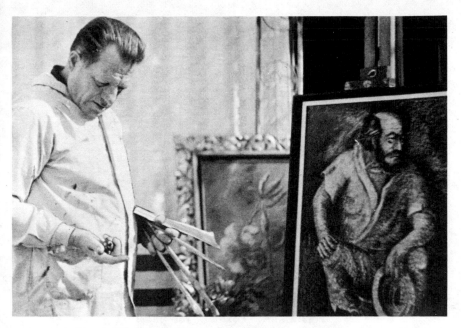

Figure 17. Artist using Magic Reflex Massager to strengthen hand.

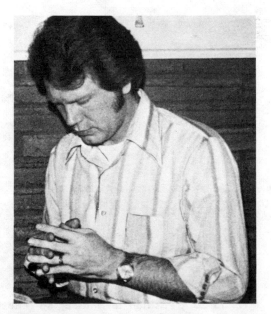

Figure 18. Position for massaging reflexes in fingers to relieve tension.

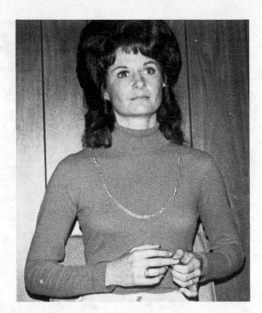

Figure 19. Position for massaging end of finger #3 to stimulate right eye, teeth, etc. on meridian line 3.

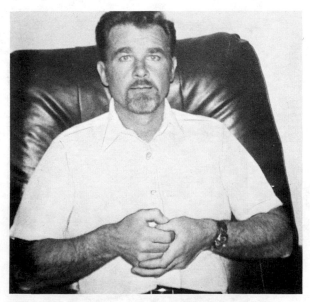

Figure 20. Position for massaging reflexes to the neck and also for headache.

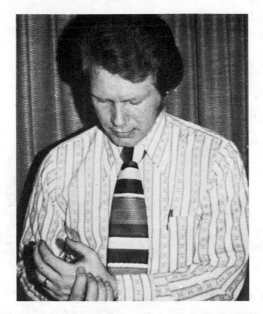

Figure 21.   Position for massaging the reflexes to the back.

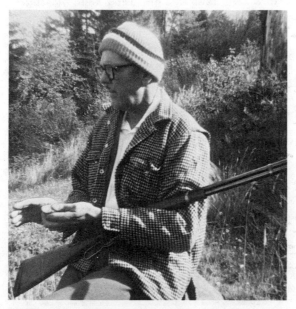

Figure 22.   Hunter massaging reflexes in the thumb to relieve tension and headache.

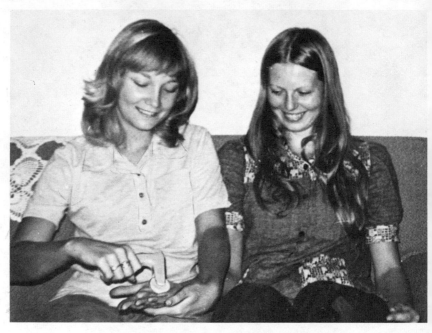

Figure 23. Teen-age girl using Rollo Massager to stimulate reflexes in friend's hand.

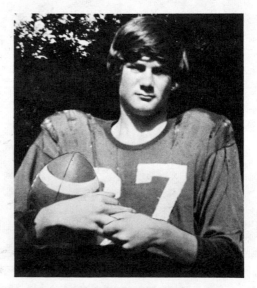

Figure 24. Football player massaging fingers to relax tension before game.

3

How to Analyze
Zone Chart No. 1

Although there are an estimated 800 to 1,000 reflex points in the body, the main ones seem to follow along certain meridian lines, from the toes to the fingers. To make it a little easier for you to locate these reflexes, study the lines on the Zone Therapy Chart #1.

You will notice how line #1 goes down the center of the body, then extends on down the inside of the leg, ending at the tip of the big toe. It also crosses over the top of the shoulder and on down the top part of the arm to the end of the thumb.

The next line, #2, is a little to the left and to the right of line #1—it also extends down the body to the second toe which we call toe #2. Notice how line #2 follows down the arm from the shoulder and ends at the tip of the second finger, etc.

All along these lines are reflex points that affect the part of the body on or near that line, which reflexologists call "zones." You can see how pressure on the big toe or thumb will affect pain in any part of line #1.

Notice how line #1 goes down through the center of the head, then the nose, mouth, neck and throat, and how it extends on down the spine, then the inside of the legs through the ankle reflexes and on down to the big toe. Notice also how it crosses over at the shoulders and comes out at the thumb, leaving a line of reflex points the full length of the arm.

See how each line follows through a definite part of the body.

Line 1: Pain in any part of Zone or line #1 may be treated and overcome, temporarily at least and often permanently, merely by exerting pressure on the thumb or the big toe.

Line 2: Then we follow line #2 down through the head, the corner of the eye, the nose, the teeth, side of the neck, etc., on down through the body to the second finger and second toe.

Line #3: Note how line #3 is a little farther over to the side of the head, through the middle of the eye and follows on down through the body, ending at finger #3 on the hand and toe #3 on the foot.

Line 4: now look at line #4 as it moves over near the outer edge of the head and moves on down the body to the leg and on down to the fourth toe; traveling down the arm and ending at the fourth finger tip.

Line #5: Notice how line #5 goes down through the ear, the outer side of the face, following on down the outer side of the body to the little toe, and down the under side of the arm to the end of the little finger.

You can see how the flow of this vital life energy is stimulated in different areas as you press on a certain toe or finger or a reflex point in the hand.

A firm pressure on the thumb will flow down the meridian line #1 and will control all the points along this line. You can see how any congestion along any one of these lines could cause trouble in another part of the body.

You can see how eye troubles can be helped by pressure exerted on the second, third and fourth fingers, and as we follow on down the hand, how internal organs are stimulated by pressure and massaging of certain reflexes in the hands, such as the stomach, kidneys, intestines and colon, etc. See Chart #2 and run an imaginary line down the body on this chart.

This is why you can help the deaf to hear by working on the fourth and fifth fingers, and why you can stop a toothache by anesthetizing it with pressure on the fingers which are in the same zone as the aching tooth. If it were the front tooth, you would use pressure on the thumb and the finger next to it, etc. This will be more fully explained in a forthcoming chapter on teeth.

I am giving you this zone chart to help you understand better how this wonderful method of pressing on a certain point in your hands or feet works for your benefit, and to make it easier for you to find the reflexes to the part of the body you are interested in helping. You can see the simplicity of how a firm stimulating pressure on certain reflex points in the hands, fingers, feet, and toes controls individual zones.

The vertical lines that I have been explaining to you are merely the *clues* to help you locate specific reflexes to certain glands and organs, as they travel across the network of channels of your body.

Do not be discouraged if they seem a little complicated at first. Just keep referring to them, and before you know it, they will all be fixed in your mind. This is very important because there will be many occasions when you will be away from home and not have your book with you just when you need it.

4

Reflexology Versus Acupuncture

Considerable publicity has been given recently in the press to the Chinese method of treating illness with "acupuncture." Reflexology and acupuncture come from an ancient art of healing.

They are related and based on the same principle of healing. Where the Chinese insert needles in certain points of the body, we of the western world use our fingers to press these vital stimulating points in the hands and the feet with like results of activating the vital life force:—thus, sending instant healing forces to malfunctioning parts of the body, even though they be far removed from the points which are being massaged, in complete safety.

Acupuncture was viewed by our former First Lady Mrs. Nixon on her visit to China, and she was quite impressed. The doctors told Mrs. Nixon, "We treat the body as a whole, while western medicine treats the symptoms. They don't get at the cause and it's a vicious, never ending circle."

The acupuncture doctors claim that there are 720 acupuncture points that all doctors learn and 180 more that are secret and known only to the masters! "That is why" we are told, "unlicensed acupunctures are so dangerous." "One misplaced needle can kill."

Health Is in Your Hands

As I explained in my previous book on Foot Reflexology, there is no portion of your wonderfully constructed feet which does not have its part to play in this reflex massage. I will say the same for your even more important wonderfully constructed hands. They, also, give you a unique way to health through the use of reflex massage.

WHAT REFLEXOLOGY IS

"Zone Therapy is scientific, subjectively and objectively," says W. D. Chesney, M.D. "That is to say that a patient using zone therapy (reflexology) knows he is getting results, and others see that he has improved.

There is no substitute, and never will be a substitute for the trained eye, ear, nose, and the sense of touch—the fingers. It is mainly with the fingers that the healer palpates as well as exerts them in zone therapy (reflexology). In medical school I learned the salient facts about reflexology. That is, that stimulation in one part of the human body often produced symptoms at far distant areas."

By using our fingers to search out and press on certain reflex buttons in the hands and the feet, we are learning to apply a simple and harmless method of healing—a method that can stop pain in all parts of the body almost instantly, with no physical or psychological harm of any kind.

REFLEXOLOGY CAN BE USED BY ANYONE

Reflex massage can be used safely by anyone, from small children to the very elderly. I know of several quite young children who are experts in giving a reflex treatment with very good results.

I have letters from people in their 70's and 80's who are not only using reflex technique on themselves with great benefit, but also on others. Can you imagine the joy of these senior citizens when they can actually help stop the pain of their ailing friends; to watch their faces as their suffering subsides after a few minutes of pressing tender reflex buttons on their hands! The relief they feel in knowing how to stop their own pains as soon as they feel them coming on, and in knowing that in many cases they are putting an end to the cause of the pain forever, with no more need of drugs or medication! What a wonderful world this will be when everyone learns how to use the marvelous magic of healing reflexology!

Chinese Acupuncture Healing
Versus Finger Reflexology

The world is looking to Chinese acupuncture at the present time. It seems that everyone is getting into the picture of sticking needles into people who are ready to turn to anything or anyone for help in their despair of suffering from all kinds of diseases and ailments which the conventional doctors can't seem to cure. When will they learn to use our safe western style of pressing these reflexes with the fingers instead of with needles, with the same results when used according to the simple directions given in this book?

Doctor Frank Moyo says:

> We are gravely concerned over the premature application of acupuncture to Americans for the relief of pain during surgery. A potentially valuable technique that has been developed over thousands of years in China is being hastily applied with little thought to safeguards or hazards. If acupuncture is applied indiscriminately, severe trauma (shock) could result in certain patients.

While Chinese medical men have expressed caution against premature use of *acupuncture,* our medical experts have used and recommended the use of *reflexology* to everyone. They have even taught their patients to use it on themselves with the full knowledge that there was no danger or harmful effects from the use of these techniques.

Reflexology Not Subject to
Man-Made Restrictions

In *A Lecture Course to Physicians,* George Starr White, M.D., writes, "A *real physician* will not hesitate to use any method that will relieve the sick. A *real quack* is one who will hesitate to use or recommend any method to relieve the sick, unless it is sanctioned by some governing board."

Giving a man a license to "heal the sick" does not make him a *physician.* Christ was a TRUE PHYSICIAN and the Bible record shows that *He did heal the sick.* Records do not show that His license was given by a power higher than God.

What A Medical Doctor Had to Say About Reflexology

Edwin Bowers, M.D., a well-known medical critic and writer, after a long, thorough investigation wrote a popular article regarding Doctor Fitzgerald's work in order that the public might be made aware of the new method of ridding themselves of pain. He called it *"Zone Therapy."* Today we call it *Reflexology.*

He wrote, "The fact that today Zone Therapy is probably known more widely throughout the United States and all places where magazines and newspapers are printed than any other single method of therapy, proves that the foundation of the work is solid."

He wrote later, "One of the most disgraceful blots on the pages of organized medicine, or what is popularly known as 'The Medical Trust,' is the fact that they have apparently, in every way possible, tried to hinder the spread of the gospel of Zone Therapy. Because it was likely to educate the people into methods of *self-treatment,* they became alarmed and in various ways they have heaped abuse upon those who practice this method." And so it is today.

Doctor Uses Reflexology as an Analgesic in Minor Operations

Doctor Bowers gives us more information by telling us how pressure on the little finger made the pinna (ear) so insensitive that pins could be put through it without any particular discomfort; how pressure on the toes served as an analgesic for minor operations around the genitals, and how pressure on the thumb, first, and second fingers was used while extracting foreign bodies from the eye without the patient even winking.

WHY REFLEXOLOGY WORKS TO BRING HEALTH BENEFITS

We are so conditioned to the need for pills, surgery, and special treatments for ailments, that many people are somewhat skeptical about the effectiveness of such a simple method as reflex massage. There are, of course, any number of theories about how or why it does work.

For instance, we are told by Alice Bailey that the "esoteric" body is really a network of fine channels which are component parts of one interlacing fine cord, one portion of this cord being the magnetic link which unites the physical and "astral" bodies, and which is broken at the time of death. This etheric web, of which we are a part, is composed of the intricate weaving of this vitalized "cord."

Thus we can easily see why massaging the reflexes to help nature open channels of health to any and all parts of the body is so positive, and why it cannot fail if applied properly. Reflexology not only helps nature open up these channels when congested *but also sends a supply of "prana," the magnetic vital life force of the universe charging through these channels like healing shock waves.* No wonder we have instant relief in so many cases of pain!

As this vital flow circulates through this network of channels, we learn that the spleen is of the utmost importance (which we will discuss further in another chapter).

Reflexology and Acupuncture

The Chinese using acupuncture and their knowledge of the thousand reflex points, tell us they do not know how or why they get results when they stick needles in certain parts of the body. No doubt the needles exert pressure on reflexes. But, my question is, why risk infection or perhaps injury at the hands of an unskilled practioner when it is not necessary? Reflexology, for all its simplicity, is a safer, more effective system for curing ailments, and carries no risk. It can be used by anyone, anywhere.

Conditions Requiring Other Types of Therapy

Of course, there may be acute conditions that require the services of a chiropractor or a medical doctor, as in the case of wounds, fractures, infections, certain diseases requiring special medications, etc., and the reader is cautioned to seek such professional help when the need is apparent.

The Basic Simplicity of Reflexology

I hope you can see the simplicity of using reflexology and why it has to give some benefit to everyone who uses it, as it stimulates the *Golden Cord of Life* within you.

All of nature's ways are simple to use once we understand them.

5

Technique of Massaging Reflexes in the Hands and Fingers

The technique of massaging these reflexes is to use the thumb or the fingers to press into the flesh over the reflex which you are trying to stimulate. You will press the thumb or the fingers into the flesh deeply enough to feel the bone or muscles underneath. *You do not rub the skin.*

You may use a press and roll movement on one spot, or a press and pull motion, as you "walk" your thumb over the hand, searching out sore spots. You will be amazed at how many you will find. Massage each spot a few minutes, and move on.

Keep the spots in mind and return to them often as you are giving yourself a treatment, except for the reflexes to the vital organs located in the center of the hands, which should be massaged according to instructions under their separate chapters.

To use another technique of massaging the reflexes in the hands, look at Figure 5-1. You will see how the thumb is pressed into the center of the palm, while at the same time the fingers are digging into the reflexes on the back of the hand. This method also stimulates a renewed flow of electrical life force throughout many parts of the body. Massage tender reflexes in back of hands as well as the palms.

HOW TO USE REFLEX TECHNIQUE ON THE HANDS

You have studied the charts and have a general idea of how

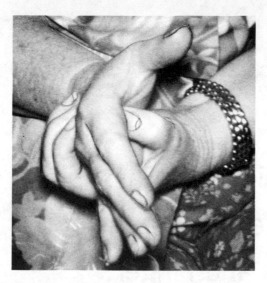

Figure 5-1. Position for pressing fingers into reflexes in the back of the hand.

each part of your body has a corresponding reflex located in the hands and fingers.

It will be best for you to sit in a relaxed position in a comfortable chair while learning to use this reflex massage on the hands and fingers.

You will find that the fingers are very important in the massaging of the reflexes as they particularly seem to control the nerves and the mentality. (See Chart #2.)

In explaining how to massage the various reflex points for the corresponding areas in the body, I will try to make it easier for you to understand by following on down through Charts #1 and #2.

We will start with the top of the head and the corresponding reflexes in the thumb, and progress down through the body, explaining the reflex to each gland and organ as we go.

Reflexes in the Thumb Stimulate Head Area

As explained earlier, reflexes in the thumb (and other areas of the hand) correspond to certain areas of the body; the left thumb stimulates the left side of the head, and the right thumb the right side of the head. For this reason, it is important to study the charts and learn which glands and organs are located on each side or in the center so that the corresponding reflexes can send their revitalizing forces directly to any ailing gland or organ.

Starting with the upper end of the thumb, you will notice that it stimulates the head area, and especially the reflexes to the pituitary gland, the most important gland of the endocrine system.

Reflexes to the Nerves, Neck and Throat

On the sides of the thumb we will find the reflexes to the nerves as in the other fingers. Where the thumb fastens on to the hand we find the reflexes to the throat and neck.

If you will take the thumb between the fingers of the opposite hand and roll it around and around, it will be the same as if some one took your head in his hands and gently rolled it from side to side. You will feel the muscles in your neck and upper back relaxing as you do this. Be sure and rotate the thumbs on both hands.

Stimulation of the pituitary gland often means a new lease on life for young and old.

Because of its close proximity, you will also be massaging the reflex to the pineal, and, of course, the brain and other areas of the head.

How to Massage the Tip of the Thumb

To start the massage of the thumb, roll the nail of the opposite thumb across the top of the thumb at its very tip, immediately under the nail, being careful not to bruise the flesh under the nail itself. This would be the palm side.

Next, take the thumb between the thumb and #2 finger of the opposite hand, and drop down to the pad which is located between the first joint and the nail, and press deeply into it with the edge of the thumb. You may get better results by using a reflex device, such as the Hand Reflex Massager shown in Figure 5-2, or any blunt instrument that will help press more firmly into the reflex buttons. Be sure to cover the whole pad with the pressing, rolling motion.

Now work the edge of your thumb on around to the back (or topside) of the thumb just below the nail, and massage this whole area clear down to the second joint. Search out any and all tender spots and massage them for a few seconds. Continue on down the sides of the thumb below the first joint, massaging as you go.

Now massage this area thoroughly on all sides, especially on the back of the thumb just below the nail.

You are sending nature's healing forces to the pituitary and pineal glands, and also to the brain and other areas of the head.

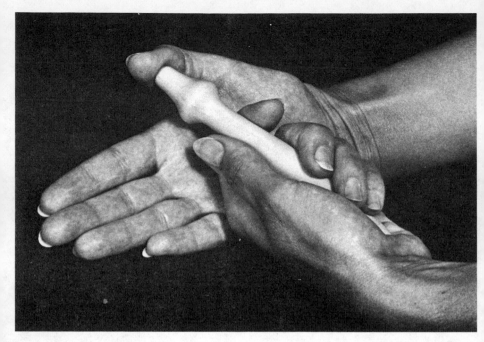

Figure 5-2. Massaging the reflexes to the pituitary and pineal glands, using the hand massager.

How to Massage for Nerves

Note on the chart that the next area says, "Nerves." Continue working on down the thumb in the same manner as above, pressing and rolling deep enough so that you can feel the solidness of the muscle and bone underneath. The nerve reflexes can be made to bring about anesthesia to deaden pain, without drugs.

How to Massage Reflexes to Throat and Neck

You will note on the chart that the next location of reflexes affects the throat and neck. Do not neglect any section of the thumb, no matter how small or insignificant it may appear to you.

Only by reaching all the reflexes will you get the full benefits of reflex massage.

Now repeat the massage of the other thumb in the same manner.

By this time you should actually feel your body responding and renewing its vital forces, and the muscles of your neck relaxing as if by magic.

Reflexology to Cure Stiff Neck

A retired friend who had fallen into the habit of falling asleep while reading, invariably woke up with a stiff neck due to faulty posture. She quickly learned from me how to massage the stiffness away by massaging the thumbs, and obtained immediate relief.

Some Reflex Buttons Are Difficult to Locate

Because we use the hands all day long, the reflexes may be more difficult to locate than in the big toe or the foot where the reflexes are protected by shoes and walking on soft surfaces such as rugs, lawns, smooth pavement, and so forth.

For this reason, I will explain the use of several helpful devices in another chapter which will enable you to massage the reflexes in the hands more conveniently. (See Chapter #8 Home Devices.)

If such devices are not immediately available, just follow the simple instructions for hand massage throughout this book, using your fingers and thumbs, nature's own "tools" for achieving and maintaining perfect health.

Study Chart #1

To get a better picture of how to locate the reflexes to certain glands, it will help if you study *Zone Chart #1* and the chapter explaining how to use it.

Practice Makes Perfect

It may take a little practice to catch onto the most effective method and the most convenient and comfortable for you.

Your health is truly in your wonderful hands if you will take time to turn the Magic Key of Reflexology as given in this book.

REFLEXES IN FINGERS STIMULATE HEAD AREA

Now let us go over the other fingers, starting with the index finger, #2, going over it slowly, beginning at the tip, which the chart indicates holds the reflexes to the sinuses.

Since the sinuses affect several areas in the head, you can readily see how the reflexes in the tips of the fingers will also affect the head in these areas.

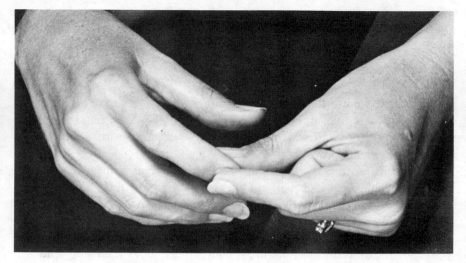

**Figure 5-3. Shows position for massaging the
reflexes on the front and back of the fingers.**

One of the best ways to massage these sinus reflexes in the tips
of the fingers is to roll the thumb nail over them just at the edge
of the nail, as you did on the thumb or first finger (#1). When you
do this correctly, you will usually feel a tender sensation as if you
are pressing on slivers in the tips of the fingers.

Roll the right thumb on the tips of the left fingers and use the
left thumb to roll along the tips of the right fingers.

Massaging Reflexes on Fingers #2 and #3

Now take finger #2 between your thumb and finger, working all
around it by pressing on the back and front of the finger (See
figures 5-3 and 5-4), searching for tender spots as you massage on
down toward the hand, as you did before. When you get to the web
between the thumb and index finger, pinch and massage it also.
When you do find a tender spot, work on it a few seconds, then go
on to the next finger, which will be the third, or middle, finger. Give
this finger the same treatment.

Keep looking at Charts #1 and #2 to see which parts of the

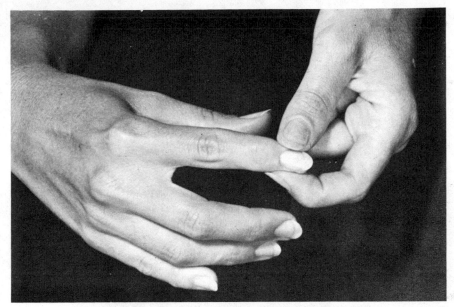

Figure 5-4. Shows position for massaging the reflexes on the side of the fingers.

body the reflexes on these fingers will stimulate. More will be given on this throughout the book.

How to Massage Fingers #4 and #5

The fourth finger is commonly called your ring finger, and the reflexes in it are very important to the outer side of your body, especially the ears, as you will read in another chapter later on.

The little finger, #5, is also important to the outer edge of your body as you can see by looking at the charts in the front of this book, and at Figure 5-5.

Be sure to massage all the fingers on both hands so that forceful life pulsations may be manifested into all of the glandular regions of your body.

HOW TO MASSAGE THE HANDS

Now let us take each reflex in the hand as you see it in your Charts No. 2 and No. 3, using the Zone Chart #1 as a guideline through the body charts, thus making it easier for you to find which reflexes stimulate certain parts of your body.

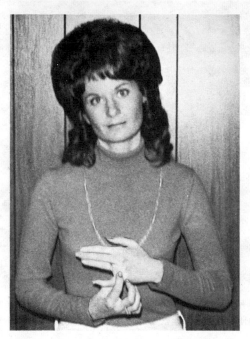

Figure 5-5.   Position for massaging reflexes to left wisdom tooth and outer ear.

How to Massage Reflexes for Eyes and Ears

Let us look just below the fingers where it will say "ears" and "eyes", with the thumb of the opposite hand you will press on the pad just about where the fingers are fastened to the hand. Use a press and pull motion here as you search out tender spots, and when you find a sore spot, keep massaging it for a few minutes to release a flow of electrical life force into the congested area, thus giving nature a helping hand in healing whatever the malfunction might be. This will be true in all cases where you find a tender spot on any reflex. Our therapy indicates: "If a reflex hurts, rub it out." (See Figures 8 and 13 in the front of the book.) Any sore spot on a reflex indicates malfunctioning of some part of your body, no matter how remote it may be from the reflex being massaged.

Nature's Gift to Relieve Pain

We do not claim that reflexology is a panacea for every ailment, but neither is any other method. Nature has given us this marvelous gift with which we can relieve pain and suffering and bring renewed health to the body and we should make use of it in every way possible. In reflexology we find a safe natural way to health and the techniques are so simple and harmless they can be used by anyone.

Reflexology Stimulates Lungs

Next, you will massage the reflexes to the lungs which are located on the pads of your hand lying under the base of the fingers. With the thumb of the opposite hand, massage along this area with the press and pull motion as explained above. It may be easier for you to massage both hands as we move along. Don't ever give yourself only half a treatment by neglecting to massage one of your hands. You can see on your chart how this would stimulate only one side of your body and neglect some of the glands and organs on the untreated side.

How to Use Reflexology for Stomach

Let us move on to the stomach reflexes which, as you can see on your chart, are located in the soft area just in front of the thumb a little below the web. You will massage this area with the thumb of the opposite hand using the press and pull motion or the rolling motion, whichever feels best to you. You will learn more of this in a forthcoming chapter on the stomach.

Reflexes to Solar Plexus

Now let us move to the center of the palm. Chart No. 2 shows that the solar plexus is located just above the stomach on the *body chart* and the reflex is shown just above the adrenal on the *hand chart*. This is where we run into congestion of the reflexes and it will be almost impossible to massage one without sending some of the current of vital life force surging through other close lying glands and organs.

Reflexology for the Thyroid

In Figure 5 in the front of book, you will see how the thumb is pressed into the reflex to the thyroid gland just on the inside edge of the large bone of the thumb. You will massage all along this area and to reach the parathyroids you will press a little deeper, as explained in the chapter on thyroid.

Where to Find the Adrenal and Kidney Reflexes

Next, we find the reflexes to the adrenal and the kidney located in the very center of the hand; see in Figure 7 in the front of book, how the thumb is held in position to massage these two reflexes. You will also learn more about these glands in another chapter.

Reflexes to Liver and Heart and Spleen

You will notice on the right hand that by moving the thumb over onto the pad under the little finger, you will be on the reflexes to the liver. If you are massaging the left hand, you will use the same position under the little finger and be on the reflex to the heart and just a little below it you will find the reflex to the spleen.

Gall Bladder, Appendix and Pancreas Reflexes

On the right hand in the same location will be the reflex to the gall bladder and appendix and the pancreas.

Across the center of the hands you will see the colon reflexes. On down toward the wrist are the reflexes to the intestines and the bladder. Notice how the thumb is held on these reflexes as shown in Figure 2 in the front of the book.

If devices other than the fingers are used, such as the Magic Massager or the Rollo Reflex Massager, then the forceful life pulsations will be manifested in all of these glandular regions at once instead of just one at a time. The use of the helpful reflex devices are explained in a later chapter in this book. (See Figures 11 and 23 in the front of the book.)

Reflexology and the Lower Lumbar Area

Now, let us look at the reflexes to the lower lumbar area. As you can see by looking at your Chart #2, they are located mostly on the wrist. See how the thumb is placed for the lower lumbar in Figure 37-3; and in Figure 37-1, the thumb is pressing on the reflexes to the prostate, uterus and penis just under the base of thumb on the palm side of the hand. In Figure 37-2, you see the thumb placed on the reflexes to the lower lumbar, the testes and the ovaries on the side of the little finger, No. 5. (See Chapter 37 on Sex Glands.) You will press in with the thumb and use the rolling motion or the press and pull method to massage these reflexes.

Importance of Lymph Glands

While we are still on the wrist, turn the hand over and on the back of the wrist, you will find the reflexes to the lymph glands. Use the same technique with the thumb—massage clear across the back of the wrist several times as the lymph glands can always stand a little natural help in their work of taking care of any infections that might invade the body.

6

Massaging the Web to Stimulate Many Parts of the Body

The webs between the fingers have many important reflexes which you will find by taking the web between the first finger and the thumb of the opposite hand and pinching and massaging it. Since this web is larger then the webs between the other fingers, we find that the reflexes in it cover a larger area of the body. See Chart #2. Pinch and massage this web thoroughly from the thin part back into the thicker area close to the hand. You will be surprised at the tender spots you will find here. Now change hands using the same pinch and roll technique, to massage the web on opposite hand being sure to cover the whole area. (See Figure 6-1.)

In this web we find the reflexes not only to the throat and neck, but also to spine, stomach, the thyroid and other internal organs, even to stimulating the liver on the reflex of the right hand web, and the heart on the reflexes in the left hand web.

Evangelist of Oral Roberts Treated by Dr. Fitzgerald

Dear Mrs. Carter:

It really made me feel good to read your letter and to know that you too were a Christian. You wound up your letter by saying "May God continue to bless you". I am 82 years old and still going strong. A Trustee of Oral Roberts Evang. Association and his University, and an International Director of the Full Gospel Business Men's Fellowship International.

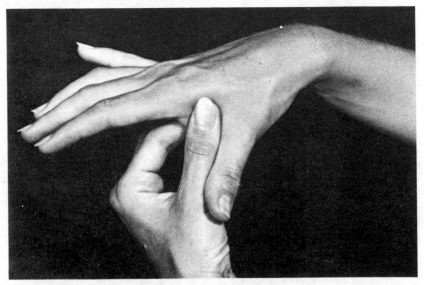

Figure 6-1. Position for massaging the re-flexes in the web of the hand.

I knew Dr. Fitzgerald of Hartford, Connecticut. He was one of the most patient men I ever knew. He knew that he had made a discovery (Zone Therapy) and took a lot of time to work it out.

I remember many years ago I had to have an operation on an Inguinal Hernia and I wanted to try out Zone Therapy. The only Anesthetic I had was a little Novocaine in my side. I applied pressure on the very ends of my fingers on the operating table. And while the operation was not absolutely painless, I was able to stand it. The novocaine was most ineffective. I also remember that I had some pain somewhere. I do not remember where. I could not find the pressure zone as he called it at the time. He said "Look in the web between the third and fourth fingers," and sure enough there it was. I could hardly touch it. And it was the same between the corresponding toes. I am a D.D.S. Past President of Hartford Dental Society, Conn. State Dental Assoc. and also N. England Dental Society. With Kindest Regards and I know God will Bless you, too. In His wonderful and powerful Name. John F. Barton

Dr. J. F. Barton

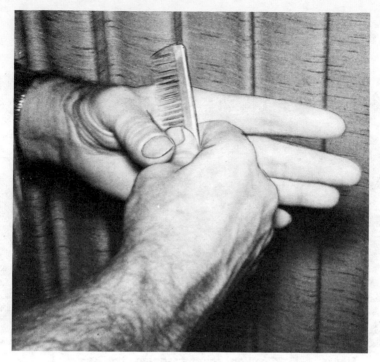

Figure 6-2. Shows teeth of reflex comb pressed into web.

USING A COMB TO MASSAGE THE WEB

Note in Figure 6-2, how the comb is held in position while exerting pressure on the web between the first and second finger. All of the webs have reflexes to certain parts of the body, and it is important to search for tender spots in the web between each finger on both hands when you are giving yourself a treatment. When you find these sore spots, massage them for a few seconds, remembering that in this way you are stimulating a current of the life force into a congested area of the body even though you may not know exactly where it is located.

We find in many cases it is more convenient merely to hold a steady pressure on certain reflexes instead of the massaging motion, with just as good results as in Figure 3 in the front of the book.

This is why the doctors used the simple methods of rubber bands, combs, and clothespins in their practice. In this way they could instruct the patient to use the method himself to alleviate his pain and in most cases cure the disorder by himself.

Report of General Improvement

My Sister-in-Law got your book, "Helping Yourself with Foot Reflexology," and she is so happy with it. She never takes sleeping pills any more and is gaining weight, and no more pain in her legs and no more pills for elimination. I can't wait to get my book.

S.M.R.

Group Uses Reflexology for Improved Health

Thank you so very much and God Bless you, Mildred Carter, for your fine work. My group is enjoying much fine health today because of you.

Sincerely yours,
Mrs. T.T.
Can.

7

How to Use the Reflexes in the Tongue

As we already know, there are some one thousand reflex points in the body, which the Chinese and some other foreign doctors activate by sticking needles into them. But in reflexology, we feel that we can get the same results by learning where the endings to these reflexes are in the hands and the feet, and accomplish the same results by the simple process of pressing and massaging them with our fingers. There are a few reflex buttons in the mouth which seem to abate distress and to enhance stimulation to some areas in certain situations.

Dr. Fitzgerald claimed the tongue had reflexes in it which followed along the meridian lines, just as in the body. Thus No. 1 line would be down the center of the tongue with lines extending out on each side. (See Chart #1.)

But your interest is in learning how to use these reflexes to help alleviate pain and illnesses in specific situations when needed. There will be several instances throughout ensuing chapters in which this technique of stimulating the reflex in the tongue will be used. So you will want to know how to master the technique of how to activate these reflexes.

How Entertainers Use Reflexology to Keep Their Voices Beautiful

First let us learn the art of pulling the tongue out as far as possible. Take a clean cloth between the fingers, stick the tongue out, then take hold of it using the cloth to hold it firmly. Now pull it out as far as possible, then move it slowly from one side to the other for a few minutes. This method of reflexology is used by many of our great entertainers, including singers, to help keep their voice beautiful. It eases throat tension, and frees the voice. It is a help in stopping a sore throat and even a cold. In this way you are employing stimulation to the first, second, and third meridian lines, the region which governs the function of the vocal chords, the larynx, and the respiratory passages, and is helpful where there is illness caused by malfunctioning in this area.

How to Press Reflexes in the Tongue

Next we will learn how to press down on the tongue farther back in the mouth for added stimulation in specified cases which you will learn more about in following chapters. To reach the reflexes farther back on the tongue, some kind of a probe will have to be used. The handle of a table knife or of a spoon will do, if you don't have a tongue probe. Press down on the back of the tongue as hard as you can stand, hold it for two or three minutes at a time. If it causes gagging, start closer to the mouth and work back a little at a time. This technique will be given in subsequent chapters so learn it well.

You will recognize that you are stimulating the reflexes on the same zone as the thumb is on. If you move it over a bit you will be on the zone with the next fingers, etc. This is an added stimulation to any part of the body which is on the first, second, and third zones.

If you are unable to find a tongue probe on the market Stirling Enterprises, in Cottage Grove, Oregon will probably have them.

You will be amazed at the tender spots you will find in your tongue as you use this pressure in different places. It can be used in conjunction with pressure on the reflexes in the first, second, and third fingers, for added stimulation of the electrical life force in this particular area of the body where the meridian zone lines pass through. (See Chart #1.)

8

How to Use Home Devices
to Relieve Pain

When Dr. Fitzgerald first started using pressure on the reflexes to alleviate pain and cure many diseases, he discovered how to make use of several devices found in the kitchen, to help him hold a steady pressure for a prolonged period of time in order to anesthetize certain parts of the body, in cases of toothache, earache, labor pains, and many other painful ailments.

By putting pressure on the tips of certain fingers and holding it a few minutes he found that he could deaden the part of the body to which the reflex went. So to save his time, he found that the ordinary clothespin would work even better then his fingers, and be a lot less tiring. He found that he could also have his patient keep up the treatment at home with this simple ingenious device.

Next he devised the idea of wrapping rubber bands around the fiingers, which served the same purpose by holding pressure on certain reflexes in the fingers to anesthetize other parts of the body.

He also found that the teeth of a comb worked best in many situations, as the comb could be used to hold pressure on several reflexes at a time, not only on the fingers, but on all parts of the hands, and this simple method could also be used safely at home when needed.

There is the small rubber ball which is still used by many doctors, and in many hospitals as therapy for victims of arthritis, stroke, and various other kinds of paralysis.

All through this book you will see many illustrations and directions on the use of several improved reflex devices which have been designed especially for reflexology. These may be obtained at local markets, or from Stirling Enterprises, Inc., Cottage Grove, Oregon.

It is not essential that you have these reflex devices to obtain beneficial and lasting results when using reflex massage. Reflexology is a natural way to health, and the natural use of your fingers will work wonders in releasing the universal flow of the vital life force to send it surging through all the channels of your body, bringing you renewed health and vitality. You will be given directions on how to use reflex massage with the fingers as well as the devices in the following chapters.

The aforementioned reflex devices are especially beneficial in holding a steady pressure when needed in certain areas of the body.

HOW YOU CAN USE COMBS TO RELIEVE
PAIN AND REGAIN HEALTH

Pressing and massaging the reflexes in the hands with the fingers will give satisfactory results most of the time, but there will be certain cases where a steady pressure will be needed for several minutes at a time. This is where the value of using the comb technique comes in.

Any type of comb may be used in an emergency, but keep in mind that most combs are made of plastic and could very easily break and injure the hands or fingers if too much pressure were placed on the teeth. The doctors recommended that a metal comb be used in zone therapy for this reason, and also because the vibrations of the metal were thought to help in stimulation of the life forces.

It is a known fact that certain metals do give off "rays" or "vibrations" that stimulate the current of life forces in the body. Scientific studies are now being made regarding metal therapy.

Pressure on the reflexes using the metal comb is very helpful as it reaches several reflexes in the hands at one time, thus being more effective than massaging just one reflex at a time.

You will note in Figure 8-1 how the teeth of the comb are used to press into the palms of the hands for special uses as explained in other chapters. In Figure 8-2 you see the tips of the fingers being pressed onto the teeth of the comb while the thumb is pressing on the end of the comb. The teeth of the comb can be used in the webs between the fingers. Also, the back of the comb may be used for a firm steady pressure when needed.

You will learn methods of using the comb technique to help in relieving pain and illnesses of varying types in following chapters.

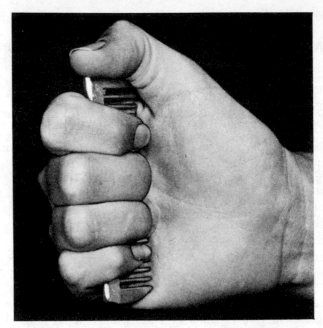

Figure 8-1. Pressing teeth of comb into the palm of the hand.

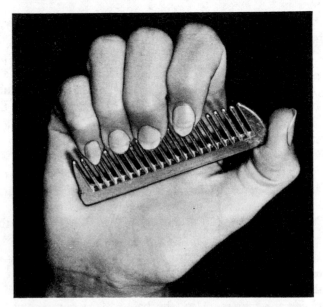

Figure 8-2. Pressing teeth of comb into finger tips.

Using Comb Technique for Instant Vitality

Take the comb in your hand and press the teeth into the tips of the fingers, now press the thumb on the end of the comb as shown in Figure 8-2. If you have two combs, use them both, one in each hand, for a vitalizing sensation of renewed life-force surging through your whole body.

Now try moving the teeth of the comb on different locations of the fingers. Try pressing the teeth into the first finger on all sides, remembering also to press the thumb on the end of the comb, as this stimulates the two important endocrine glands, the pituitary and the pineal. Thus you are giving different parts of the body currents of vital life force with the added stimulation of the King glands at the same time. Why shouldn't you feel a renewed exhilaration of health almost instantly? Use this method on all the fingers.

This is instant vitality at your finger tips. As you press the teeth of the comb into certain reflexes, a stimulated flow of vital energy is sent surging through your body to the areas corresponding with the reflexes being pressed.

Using Comb to Locate Reflex Trouble Spots

Next, press the teeth of the comb into the palm of your hand. Press it into different areas holding it in each position for a few seconds to get the feel of it. You will notice in Figure 8-1 how the comb presses into several reflexes at the same time. In using this method of massage it is easy to search out the trouble spots in your body. As you press the teeth of the comb into the palm of your hand you are able to stimulate several parts of the body at the same time. By checking on Chart #2, you will be able to tell which areas in the body are sending out distress signals as you feel tenderness in certain reflexes.

Comb for Web Reflexes

Now take the comb in one hand and press the teeth into the webs between the fingers of the opposite hand; move it around and even up on the sides of the fingers. When you find sore spots, hold it a few seconds. If you find the reflexes are too tender, then use the back of the comb for a few days. Remember to massage the reflexes on both hands.

Not only will this give you a feeling of well being and vitality, it will help you become familiar with the technique of using the comb pressure massage when it is recommended in subsequent chapters.

TECHNIQUE OF USING RUBBER BANDS TO RELIEVE PAIN

The use of rubber bands on the fingers is an added help in relieving pain quickly, and in many cases, permanently. Dr. Bowers states, "This pressure therapy has an advantage over any other method of pain relief, inasmuch as it has been proved that, in contradistinction to opiates, when Zone (reflex) pressure relieves pain, it likewise tends to remove the cause of the pain, no matter where this cause originates. And this relief is often accomplished in conditions where seemingly one would not expect to secure any therapeutic, or curative results."

Note in Figure 14 in the front of the book how the rubber bands are wrapped tightly around certain places on the fingers. If you have studied your chart, you will recognize that the left side of the body is being treated because the bands are on the fingers of the left hand. As I have stated before, the fingers are the key to many parts of the body because the palm is too small to accommodate all of the reflexes located within the body.

In Figure 14, in the front of the book we see the rubber bands wrapped around the third, fourth and fifth fingers of the left hand, which we recognize from the explanation in earlier chapters stimulates the outer edge of the head and glands and organs on the left side of the body.

If the thumb, second, and third fingers are involved, we would be treating the central part of the left side of the head, and corresponding organs as explained in other chapters.

By making use of the rubber bands to keep a steady pressure on the reflex buttons, you can easily see that several reflexes can be controlled at once instead of just one reflex point at a time, as when using just our fingers to press these buttons. This makes it possible to control pain and illnesses faster and more conveniently, especially if we are too ill or in too much pain to press each reflex button for any length of time to get results. By just wrapping a rubber band around the fingers, we are able to control pain from many causes in just a few minutes. You may use whatever size band that is handy.

Wrap it around the fingers until it gives a firm pressure, but not too tight. It may be used on one or several fingers at a time.

Warning on Use of Rubber Bands

Do not leave the rubber bands on the fingers long enough for the fingers to turn blue. Be sure and take them off at the time the fingers *start* to turn blue, not *after*, as the circulation is being cut off. You can remove them for a few minutes and then put them back on again. NEVER put the rubber bands on a child or an ill person who is not mentally alert without staying with them and removing the bands *before* the fingers turn blue.

Reflex Clamps are Easier and Safer to Use

Now that the reflex clamps are on the market, you will find them safer and easier to use as they are designed to give the same benefits of anesthesia as the rubber bands without interfering with the circulation. (See Figure 10-1 and Chapter 10, "How To Use Reflex Clamps.")

How Reflexology Stopped Toothache

Before the reflex clamps were available, I developed a painful toothache and could not get into a dentist's office for at least a week. It was a back tooth on the right side, so I wrapped the three outside fingers on the right hand with rubber bands. I kept doing this off and on all day until the dentist called and said he could see me. He tapped on my teeth but to my surprise there was no pain. The X-ray showed perfect teeth. I evidently had neuralgia and the pressure on the fingers had stopped the pain. I was embarrassed about trying so hard to see a dentist. I did not tell him I was a reflexologist, but I mentioned that I had read about wrapping the fingers with rubber bands and had tried it. He wasn't even interested.

It is sad that the doctors and dentists of today are so brainwashed in what they are taught in their long years of schooling that they have lost all interest in anything that might be a natural and simple answer to many suffering patients who are unable to use opiates.

A little knowledge of reflexology could be the answer, and the technique would take only a few hours to learn.

How a Doctor Cures Breast Tumor with Reflexology

Doctor Bowers tells of a case of breast tumor, with two fairly good-sized nodes, as large as horse chestnuts. The lady had made arrangements to be operated on by a prominent surgeon in Hartford. She postponed the operation for a few weeks on account of the holidays.

Meantime, she had been instructed to make pressure on the tongue and use rubber bands on the fingers for the relief of the breast pain, which he says brought quite complete relief. When she went to make arrangements for the operation, the surgeon found the growth so reduced in size that he was unwilling to operate. The tumor has since completely disappeared.

Doctor Bowers says, "This patient and the name of the surgeon who saw her before and after are at the disposal of any physician who may regard this as untrue."

How a Uterine Fibroid Disappeared

"A small uterine fibroid made a similar happy exit, as a result of pressure made on the floor of the mouth and the regular practice of squeezing the joints of the thumb and first and second fingers.

"Lymphatic enlargments, as painful glands in the neck, armpits, or groin, yield even more rapidly to this pressure then do tumors. And while no claims are made to the effect that cancer can be cured by zone therapy, yet there are many cases in which pain has been completely relieved, and the patients freed from further use of opiates, and in a few cases the growths have also entirely disappeared."

From the files of Doctor Bowers, who is now deceased.

Reflexology a Godsend

I do not advise anyone to depend on reflexology as a cure-all, but if this simple, harmless method of applying pressure to certain areas of the hands and feet, and fingers and toes, will alleviate pain from any cause, it is a *GODSEND* for the whole human race.

The acupuncture doctors are using the same principles of stimulating this life force to anesthetize pain and heal diseases, by using needles, which we know can be quite dangerous if used by the layman or even an untrained practitioner. We can be thankful that our doctors rediscovered our western style of Reflexology by using the simple pressure method of the fingers and other harmless devices found in our homes, to accomplish like results.

9

How to Use the
Magic Massager

In my search for a simple device that would satisfactorily massage most of the reflexes in the hands, I developed an improved Palm Massager, shown in Figure 9-1, which we call the Magic Reflex Massager.

The therapy of the rubber ball has been used by doctors and hospitals for years. Patients who have arthritis in the fingers, hands,

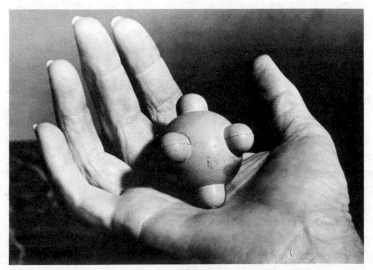

Figure 9-1. How to hold the Magic Reflex Massager.

and arms have been given a small rubber ball to hold and told to squeeze it constantly, with satisfying results.

I felt there was a need for a device that would dig in and *massage the reflexes* in the hands for even better results, so I designed a new type of massager for this purpose. The beneficial results have been even more than I had hoped for.

Case History of First Experiment with Magic Massager

When I got my first sample Magic Massager, I gave it to my husband to try on our way home. He really liked the feel of it, and kept squeezing and rolling it in one hand and then the other as he drove toward home. Suddenly he said, "I feel kind of sick." I told him to quit using the massager which he did, and the sick feeling stopped. *He had over-massaged the reflexes in his hands.* This is when we realized how powerful this little massager is!

Magic Massager Relieves Aching Arm

My son-in-law was having trouble with his arm going to sleep at night, and aching at times during the day. He tried using the Magic Massager every night as directed, for about two weeks, and has had no more trouble with his arm since. He still uses it occasionally to make sure the trouble does not return.

TECHNIQUE FOR USING THE MAGIC MASSAGER

Take the Magic Massager in one hand and close the fingers around it. Now squeeze. Notice how its little "fingers" press into several reflexes of the hand at one time. Roll it over and it will press into a different set of reflexes. Each time you roll it a little, it reaches different reflex points (see Figure 9-2.)

Do this for about two minutes, then change the massager to the other hand, again massaging for about two minutes. You will immediately feel a stimulation of magnetic vitality surging through your whole body. You will not want to lay this little Magic Massager down —but remember: *don't over-massage!* You can do it again tomorrow, or maybe later in the day if you feel O.K. after using it the first time.

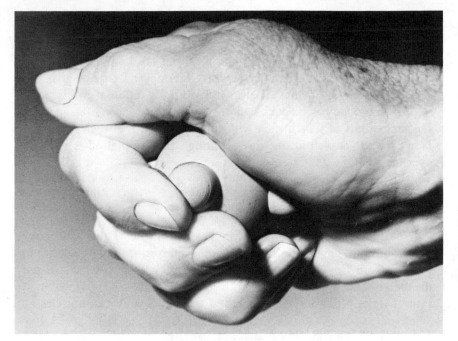

Figure 9-2.   Magic Massager used in one hand.

Magic Massager Is Safe for Anyone

There is no danger in using this massager, but it is so powerful in its stimulation of the reflexes to so many glands at once, that to release all this new life force so suddenly is a shock after they have been almost dormant for a long time. So follow directions and renew your vitality and health almost immediately.

How to Use Magic Massager in Both Hands

Take the massager and place it in the palm of the left hand, as in Figure 9-1. Now cup the right hand over the massager, clasping the fingers around each other as shown in Figure 1 in the front of the book. Roll the massager between the hands in several directions. Feel how the little "fingers" press into the reflexes of both hands simultaneously.

Due to the double action of stimulating these reflexes, you are sending the magnetic electrical force surging through the web of channels surrounding your body with a double force of healing power which you will probably feel almost immediately. So, I tell you again, *do not over-massage, at first.* You can tell how long and how often to use the massager after the first few days. I cannot give you any certain length of time, as each individual is different in his need.

If your body is in poor condition, use the Magic Massager for shorter periods of time at first with longer periods between massages. Don't try to get well in one day, although the temptation is great to over-massage.

Difference Between Magic Massager and Palm Massager

Do not confuse the Magic Massager with the "Palm Massager" which has no fingers to stimulate the reflexes. Many benefits are derived from using the palm massager, especially if you do not use the hands and arms much in your daily activities. It *can* be used several times a day to help strengthen the hands and arm muscles.

Using the Magic Reflex Massager on the Fingers and Thumbs

Take up the Magic Massager and start pressing its tiny fingers into the end of the thumb. Now press the fingers of the Magic Massager on all sides of the thumb, pressing and rolling all the way down to the base of the thumb. Use this same rolling-pressing motion on each of the other fingers.

You will be amazed at the sore spots this little magic ball will find for you in the fingers as well as in the hands. Remember our motto, *"If it is sore, work it out."* But don't try to do it the first day or even the first week. Even though Reflexology does seem to work miracles in many cases, take your time—your body was a long time getting into the condition it is now in, so don't try to shock it into perfect working order in just a few days. Give it a chance to rebuild into perfection.

The Magic Massager Useful in Sports Activities

The Magic Massager is being used in many sports activities. Golfers find that by rolling it around in their hands several times a day, it seems to improve control to swing the club just right by giving the right amount of strength to the muscles where needed, and that it leaves a feeling of relaxation and confidence when used just before a game.

Bowlers also find the Magic Massager very helpful in keeping their hands and arms strong and relaxed before a game, and to relax the fingers after the game is over.

This magic ball is popular even in the field of competitive sports of the younger generation.

How to Get Double Benefits from the Magic Massagers

After using the Magic Massager in one hand at a time for several days, you are now ready to use two Magic Massagers if you have them, using one in each hand for double benefits.

By looking at Chart #2, you can see how the reflexes to most of the organs and glands on both sides of the body will be stimulated into renewed life by the flow of the Vital Universal Energy as many of the reflex buttons are pressed in both hands simultaneously.

Take a Magic Massager in each hand and use a squeeze and press motion for a few moments, then roll it into another position and press and squeeze again, placing the fingers of the massagers into different areas as you rotate them in your hands.

You can easily see why this little massager works such magic when used as directed, when you look at Chart #2 and see how the reflexes are all crowded up into such a small area. The Magic Massager is revitalizing almost the whole body.

How to Use Reflexology to Strengthen Inner Muscles of the Body

In strengthening the hands and arms, we find another unexpected benefit. As you press with both hands on this Magic Massager, you will feel tension on every muscle in your body, especially in the inner muscles around the glands and organs. You can even feel the back muscles become tight.

Notice how the inner muscles of the lower extremities are tightened. This kind of exercise alone is worth more than a million dollars to all of us in this day of sagging inner muscles caused by the lack of natural exercise.

Think what this means in rebuilding the body. Not only is it set free of congestion by the magnetic life forces as they are sent surging through our web of channels, stimulated by massaging the reflexes, but at the same time the inner muscles are tightened and brought back to normal.

Of course, you will have to control this muscle tightening exercise in the extremities by holding the Magic Massager in both hands and pressing with a squeezing motion. This will put tension on the muscles in the upper part of your body. Now use this same pressing motion of the massager and strain the lower part of the body by pulling the muscles in and up toward your waist.

This reflex exercise of the lower part of the body will not only benefit the lower lumbar area, but also the bladder and urethral channel. It will benefit the reproductive organs to such an extent that many feel a renewed interest in their sex life, as if they have been rejuvenated, since reproductive organs are truly the organs of rejuvenation.

Warning: don't over-do this the first week, or you will become very sore and think something has gone wrong with your organs.

Do this exercise only once a day for the first two days, then increase to two times a day for two days, etc., until the muscles have adjusted. This is the same as if you over-exercised your legs or arms and got cramps in the muscles. Don't get cramps in the inside muscles. Just take it easy the first week or two and you will find yourself becoming a new and beautiful YOU, thanks to the miracles of nature, and Reflexology.

How the Magic Massager Strengthened an Artist's Hands

A very popular artist, whom I knew, was devoting his full time to painting pictures, murals in churches, and also teaching art. I noticed that he had started dropping his brush quite frequently during art classes. One day I stayed over and after everyone had left I asked him about it. A worried look came over his face and he said, "I don't know what is wrong. I just suddenly lose control of my right hand, for no reason that I know of. If I lose the use of my hand I am done. I have devoted my life to the study of art, and this is all I can do and it is the work I love."

I took one of the Magic Massagers out of my purse and showed it to him. I asked if he would try it for a while and see what it would do for him. Since he knew that I was a reflexologist and had much success with so many cases, he was delighted to take my advice and try the massager.

I told him to work it in both hands and especially the right hand every time he got a chance. The next week, when I went to class, I noticed he didn't drop his brush once.

Later he told me how grateful he was for such a simple remedy, which he claims saved not only his business, but his happiness, and also alleviated some malfunctioning in his body which might have proved serious if it hadn't been stopped. We never did know what had caused the trouble, but were more than delighted that it had vanished. This occurred several years ago and, thus far, there has been no recurrence of his trouble and he has been able to go on to even greater works of art. He says, "Thanks to the little Magic Massager," which he still uses every day. See Figure 17 near the front of the book.

10

How to Use
Reflex Clamps

When a steady pressure is held for a short period of time on a reflex, it causes an anesthesia of the corresponding part of the body. If we press the reflexes of the thumb and hold it a few moments, it not only stops pain in various parts of the head, but in most cases cures it permanently. See Figure 10-1. Perhaps we should call Reflexology a curing anesthesia. When it is used to stop pain, it also eliminates the cause of the pain. How does it do this? When these reflexes are agitated in any way, they start a vital force of energy flowing through the channels, cleansing away all congestion as they make their way through the magnetic lines which lead to the specific area to which the reflex being agitated is related.

If we put pressure on the ends of certain fingers, we will send a surge of electrical energy through the channels to different related parts of the body which will stimulate them into renewed vitality and healing, or if the pressure is held for a few minutes, it will also anesthetize an area to such an extent that it can even be operated on. A tooth can be pulled without pain; a cinder may be removed from the eye without blinking.

Chinese Use "Acupuncture"—
We Use "Reflexology"

This is all the Chinese do with acupuncture—agitate these reflexes with needles. You can get the same results by using your fingers or various harmless devices such as the reflex clamps which you can

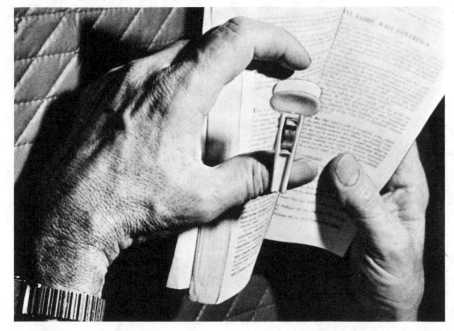

Figure 10-1. Reflex clamp being used on thumb.

place on the fingers for five or ten minutes at a time. You will read in the following chapters how even your medical doctors used this simple method of inhibiting pain in such cases as childbirth, back troubles and even operations, only they used such items as rubber bands and clothespins to hold pressure on the finger reflexes.

Look at Figure 10-2 and see how a reflex clamp is fastened on the ring finger of the left hand. Many cases of complete deafness have been cured with nothing more than this simple pressure on the end of the ring finger several times a day. Many people have been able to hear within a few minutes after the clamp has been placed on the finger. You will read in a chapter on the ears, elsewhere in this book, how many, almost unbelievable cases of the deaf regained their hearing in this way.

If you will look at Charts #1 and #2, you will see how the clamp placed on certain fingers will anesthetize the areas through which the zone line runs.

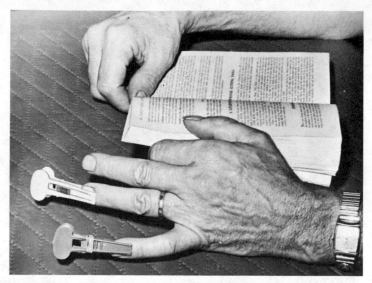

Figure 10-2. Using reflex clamps on fingers #4 and #5.

If, for instance when we put a clamp on finger 2 as in Figure 13, in the front of the book, we can see how this would affect the eyes, the nerves in that area, the head to a certain degree, and also other parts of the body. If the reflex clamps are used on the finger of the right hand, then the right side of the body will receive the benefit.

If the reflex clamps are used on the left hand, then this would affect the areas on the left side of the body.

If the reflex clamp is placed on finger No. 5, you can see by looking at Chart #1 how the meridian line runs down the outer side of the body on the same side as the clamped finger, thus stimulating the areas which this line passes through.

Doctor Demonstrates Proof of Reflexology

In his book, "A Lecture Course to Physicians," Dr. White tells us of several cases where he used pressure on the fingers to get the following results.

I was talking to a doctor friend who did not believe in Zone Therapy (Reflexology). As I was talking with him, I took hold of the thumb and the index (#2) finger of his right hand and began pressing on them, at the same time talking to him. I did not give him a hint as to what I was trying to do. After about two minutes, I stopped the pressure and took a metal applicator from my pocket and laid it on his right eyeball. He did not flinch and could not believe what I was doing. I tried laying the applicator on the other eyeball and he then understood that his right eyeball was anesthetized. I then took some steel pins that were sterilized and stuck them in his face and told him to look in the mirror. He withdrew the pins and asked when he could start studying this work with me.

The same day in the hotel, I met a lady who had a severe headache. I exerted pressure upon the fingers in the indicated zones and within five minutes the headache had disappeared. I had the same success in treating a toothache.

You will learn the technique of using the reflex clamps to treat many painful diseases and illnesses in the ensuing chapters, and the knowledge of reflexology will open up a whole new way of life, not only for you but also for others whom you will be able to free from the darkness of illness and pain when you use the magic of Reflexology.

The reflex clamps are easy to use and safe for any age.

11

Animals Show Proof That Reflexology Really Works

When people are told of the wonderful results produced by reflex massage, the first thing they say is "Oh, it is just psychosomatic (all in the mind)." Doctors who do not understand the scientific art of reflexology use this as the only answer, but when you tell them it works as well on *animals,* they have to change their minds. Animals certainly don't know what you are trying to do when you use pressure on certain reflexes to anesthetize ailing parts of their bodies.

Your Mind Can Influence Your Body

It can't be denied, however, that the power of man's mind does influence the condition of his body, but an illness that is induced by wrong thinking is not *imaginary*—it is *real*.

We are constantly reminded of all kinds of terrible diseases via TV, papers, magazines, and advertisements—consequently we are being brain-washed to be *illness prone*.

How Your Thoughts Can Control Your Future

If the mind dwells on any illness for a certain period of time, the body is being conditioned for that disease, and in a matter of time will accept what the mind has been preparing it for; and it then materializes. This is a scientific fact. We all know that our thoughts do control our future, for good or for bad, depending on how we *direct* them by conscious effort.

You Can Build a Happy, Healthy Future

As I stated in my book, *The Power of Thought*, "What you thought yesterday, you are living today; what you think today, you will live tomorrow."

Your thoughts have more power than you realize, and when you use them for health combined with the healing power of reflexology, you can live the rest of your life in the joy of perfect health.

Proof That Benefits of Reflex Massage Are Real

The following true accounts of animals treated with reflex massage are proof that the results obtained were real, not mental.

Case History of Reflexology Used on a Horse

Doctor White, an M.D., tells of how he used pressure on the reflexes of a horse in order to operate on its hip.

> Some years ago one of my horses backed into a window and got a large piece of glass into the sacral region. I tried putting her into a narrow stall and tying her legs so I could operate, as a large incision had to be made to extract the foreign body. Nothing would avail. Finally, one of my men said that if I would let him tie a slip noose, which he called a "twitch" around the horse's nose and hold it, he thought I could operate. He made this "twitch" out of a piece of small rope, put it on the horse's nose, and held it a few minutes.
>
> I thought I would have to obtain the services of a veterinarian, but told the man to put the "twitch" on again, tie it tightly, and hold it for two or three minutes. I perched on a box in a stall at one side so I would not be kicked, and to my surprise I made a large incision and took out the glass without the horse flinching.
>
> At other times I have had occasion to do minor operations on cows and pigs, and have been able to do them by putting a "twitch" on the nose, and the animals did not seem to experience any pain. In fact, they would begin to eat the moment the "twitch" was removed.
>
> I have seen young stallions castrated in this same manner without hardly flinching, and have seen the same work with young pigs. I have observed that the pressure had to be held for two or three minutes before the operation began.

Would you call this psychosomatic? The pressure on the nose anesthetized the sacral nerve as the sacral region and the nose are in the same zone on an animal.

How the Author Used Reflex Massage to Cure Her Dog of Asthma

Inky was a little black Pomeranian who was a part of the family. When he was about three years old, he started to have spells of asthma, not bad at first, just periods of wheezing for a short time every two or three weeks.

Then one Sunday, when we had a houseful of company, Inky had a bad attack, wheezing so loud he disturbed everyone and I didn't have time to try to help him.

That night after everyone had gone home, I rubbed his throat and tried to get him to smell vinegar fumes and other remedies, all to no avail. He just seemed to get worse. After we went to bed, I couldn't go to sleep because of his loud wheezing and I knew he was suffering, so I suffered with him not knowing what to do, then it came to my mind, "Why not try reflexology on him?"

I called softly to him to come over to my bed. He got out of his little box in the corner and came willingly over to me. Without getting out of bed, I rolled him over on his back on the rug and started to pinch and massage the pads on his little feet. I had no idea where to look for reflexes on an animal, so I followed our reflexology motto, "If it hurts, work it out."

First I started to pinch and press the large pad in the center of his front feet. I could tell this hurt him as he would flinch, yet he seemed to want me to keep rubbing it. I also went over the pad of every toe on both front feet in this manner, pinching and pressing and rubbing. Sometimes he would jerk his foot clear away from me but would quickly put it back into position. He knew I was doing the one thing that would help him.

I noticed that his heavy breathing had slowed down almost immediately. Then I massaged all of the pads on his two back feet, always searching for the most tender places to rub. I found that the little extra unusable toe higher up on the feet seemed to be the most sensitive when massaged.

Inky soon fell into a quiet and peaceful sleep, and so did I. I don't know how long it was until I was awakened by his heavy breathing. I snapped my fingers and in the semi-darkness I watched his little black form come quickly to my bedside. He lay down on the rug and immediately rolled over on his back with all four feet up toward me for another treatment. I massaged only a few minutes when he seemed to be free from distress. I fell asleep while rubbing his feet. The next morning he limped from one foot to the other for a few hours, but he never had another attack of asthma.

Now, these animals could not know what was being used on them, or why, so their *minds* could not have influenced the results that were obtained when the technique of reflexology was applied.

How Reflexology Saved Pet Dog from Asthma

Mrs. S. tells of her experience with her Chihuahua.

I have had asthma and heart trouble for several years with a constant cough. Someone told us to get a Chihuahua dog and keep it near me at all times and it would help. So, three years ago my son gave me a present of a darling, tiny Chihuahua puppy. I kept him in my pocket when I was working and on my lap when sitting down, and to our surprise my symptoms vanished. Then "Wee Bits" started having spells of asthma. The veterinary said there was nothing he could do for him. I just couldn't think of losing my little pet and it hurt me to see him suffer. All I could do was pray.

Then one day my daughter bought your book "Helping Yourself With Foot Reflexology," and the first thing I turned to was your experience with your little dog who had asthma. God had answered my prayer! I started rubbing "Wee Bits" feet just as you said you did to your dog. He seemed to enjoy the treatment and it was like a miracle. My little dog started to breathe normally in just a few minutes. Now all signs of his asthma attacks have stopped and he is once again healthy and full of energy. Your wonderful book saved my little dog's life. I also use the treatments on myself and all of my friends. We are all thankful to you for writing this wonderful book showing us the positive, yet simple, way to help ourselves to stay healthy nature's way.

12

Your Life and Your Endocrine Glands

Let us give our attention to the all-important endocrine glands of which there are seven or more. These glands are all interrelated and supplement and depend on each other. They are sometimes referred to as ductless, because they have no ducts and secrete their hormones directly into the blood stream. These are the glands which form the so-called endocrine system and their normal functions and development are of great importance to the well-being of every individual. See Chart #3.

I am giving you this chapter on the endocrine glands because of their influence, not only on your health, but also on your looks, your happiness and your way of life.

This system contains the pituitary gland, situated at the base of the skull and linked with the brain. It is the commander of the whole army of endocrine glands and is often called the "king" gland. The front part secretes at least six hormones. Most of them act as dispatch riders, carrying commands to the body's other ductless glands, one of which is the growth hormone that determines whether you grow into a giant or become a dwarf.

When this gland is functioning in perfect order, growth will be normal. If you have a child who is not developing as you think he should, give nature a chance to normalize the function of this gland by stimulating the reflex to the pituitary, thus giving your child a chance to grow into a normal personality. Massaging the reflex in the center of the thumb and also the big toe will bring the necessary stimulation to this gland. If it hurts, then it is surely calling for help by sending you a message that there is trouble with the commander.

Pineal

The pineal gland is still something of a puzzle. It is known that eons ago, in the long story of evolution, it was a sort of primitive eye in many animals. In its present position inside the human head, it acts within the body as a kind of organizer or harmonizer, controlling the development of the glands and keeping them in their proper range. A pathological condition of this gland strongly influences the sex glands, causing premature development of the whole system. The endocrine system is kept harmonious and effective by its normal activity. The reflexes to this gland are also located in the thumb and big toe, just a little over toward the inside of the thumb and toe.

Thyroid

The thyroid gland, which lies near the Adam's apple, is the body's chief iodine depot.

The inner activity of our system is controlled by the thyroid gland. It is responsible for preventing the retention of water, sluggishness of the tissues, and densification of the bones. The proper development and function of the sex organs also depend upon a normal and healthy thyroid. A person is either alert or dull, quick or slow, animated or depressed, to the degree of activity of his thyroid.

Thymus

The thymus gland is located roughly level with the top of the breast bone. It also is somewhat of a mystery gland since by the time we reach adolescence, the thymus gland diminishes in size and shrinks into a fatty lump. Some scientists believe that the thymus has an influence on our immunity to disease. The more the thymus is in malfunction, the more the body is subject to illness.

To massage the reflexes to the thymus, you should massage the area between the reflexes to the lungs, just below the eye and ear reflexes. The reflexes to the thymus are located in an area where they will get the benefit of massaging the reflexes to the other glands.

There is no reason to be concerned about the thymus as long as the other endocrine glands are kept in harmony with each other.

Pancreas

The pancreas is another ductless endocrine gland which is responsible for keeping your body sugar at its proper level as I have already described in a chapter elsewhere in this book.

Parathyroids

The parathyroid glands influence the maintenance of the body's metabolic equilibrium. These small glands secrete a hormone which controls the body's supply of calcium and the content of phosphorus in the bones and the blood. People whose parathyroids are not working properly may develop twitching muscles and convulsions.

In reaching the reflexes to these tiny glands, you will use the same position as you use in massaging the reflexes to the thyroid as you can see in Figure 5, in the front of the book, except you will have to reach a little deeper. A device will probably have to be used for these reflexes if you are sure they need special attention. The eraser end of a pencil may be used or one of the hand reflex massagers.

The Adrenal Glands

Your adrenal glands promote the keenness of perception, the untiring activity, the drive to action, the inner energy, the courage, the vigor, and the fervor expressed in every way. They intensify the flow of blood, its oxygenation and organizing powers.

Now you know how important healthy adrenal glands are to your health and happiness.

To massage the reflexes to your adrenal glands, place your thumb in the center of your hand as in Figure 7 in the front of the book and press and roll the thumb in a circular motion as explained in more detail in another chapter in this book.

The Gonads (sex glands)

Truly, the gonads are the most important to your happiness of all the other ductless glands in this endocrine system. The hormones secreted by these sex glands create the inner warmth in your system, preventing all tendencies toward inflexibility. They are responsible for your ability to attract people and keep their affection and for making your personality radiant and magnetic. Sparkling eyes, self reliance, and self assurance are an indication that the gonads are functioning properly.

You can see on the Endocrine Chart #3 the location of the gonads (sex glands). Although they are not in the same place in a man as they are on a woman, you will use the reflexes to both in the same area, as you can see on Chart #2. This chart shows how the reflexes to these endocrine glands are placed on the wrist of both hands on the same side as the little finger, next to the reflexes to the lower lumbar.

Remember that these gonad glands are interrelated to all of the other endocrine glands you have just been reading about. See Figure 12 in the front of the book.

Reflexology Transforms Vital Life Forces into Activity

As I have stated before, your glandular system is the transmitter of vital life-forces which are transformed into activity through the body and this is why any improper functioning of the endocrine glands can be normalized with reflex massage. Therefore, the purpose of massaging the reflexes to these glands is to enhance the life-forces and increase their circulation in glandular areas through massaging specific reflexes, thus promoting their health and efficiency.

Insufficiencies and imbalances of the endocrine glands are usually of a functional and not an organic nature. This means that the glands are intact, but they suffer from an inadequate supply of the nerve energy and nourishment derived from an improperly oxygenated bloodstream.

Reflexology a Help for Delinquent Children

Endra Devi tells us in her book, "Forever Young, Forever Healthy," of an experiment made by Dr. Rowe in the course of which he found that moroseness, bullying, disobedience, lying, thieving and vagrancy in children were often due to a faulty pituitary function. In the face of this information, if the technique of reflexology were used in the home by the entire family, we would have less child delinquency. She goes on to tell us that an increase of blood supply and nerve energy naturally improves and heightens the functional activities of the glands. I know this is true of Yoga, and it is also true that we can accomplish the same results by massaging the reflexes to these endocrine glands.

Chinese Used Gold Needles— Reflexology Uses Fingers

The Chinese also successfully used for many thousands of years a similar approach in their treatments. Instead of doing Yoga exercises, they inserted a gold or silver needle into certain vital spots in the body in order to direct uninterrupted life flow to these various parts of the body. This was the old way of doing acupuncture; today, the Chinese use many needles. In reflexology, we use only our fingers to contact and strengthen these pulsations in order to animate their activity by removing the obstructions which prevent a free flow of the vital life-force into malfunctioning parts of the body.

Reflexology Keeps Glands in Tune

Remember that reflexology deals with the functions of life and the endocrine glands are the orchestra of your life; so keep them in tune by using reflex massage and your whole being will be in harmony with the symphony of the universe.

13

Anemia Can Be Helped with Reflexology

The spleen serves as a storehouse for iron needed by the blood. Anemia is caused by lack of iron in the bloodstream, and if neglected for a long period of time, can cause serious trouble.

If you will look at Chart #2, you will see how the spleen is located on the left side, just under the heart, and the reflex to the spleen lies just below the heart reflex. If you look at Figure 18-1 (chapter on heart), you will see how the thumb is placed on the left hand just under the little finger for massaging the heart reflex. You will use this same position for massaging the reflex to the spleen, except that you will move the thumb just a bit lower toward the wrist. If you are anemic, you will have no trouble finding a tender spot here. This may be a small spot not much bigger than a pea. If it is sore, press and roll the thumb on this button until you have worked the soreness out, helping nature stimulate this lazy congested gland back into a healthy condition.

Anemic Girl Has Energy of Eighty Years

When I was very young, a doctor told me I was so anemic I had the energy of an eighty-year-old-woman. I was so tired it was an effort for me to get out of bed, let alone walk around. If you ever feel like that, massage the spleen reflex to see if you can find any tenderness. When you do, *massage it out,* and get a good supply of iron.

Remember that the spleen is the storage container of your life energy forces, so keep it in perfect condition by massaging the reflexes under the heart area on the left hand.

How a Man Regained Energy

Mr. B. writes, "About three weeks ago I became run down, no pep, no usual get-up-and-go. I had been reading about the spleen in your book on Foot Reflexology. I thought maybe that could be my trouble.

"Sure enough, the spleen reflex was very sore—so I massaged it, first day about a minute, next day a little longer. After about three days, I was my usual self. Sounds like a fairy story, but it *really worked*. Now I massage my own feet every day, thanks to Mrs. Carter, I feel great."

B. R., Calif.

"Dear Mrs. Carter:
I have already experienced a change in my body since buying your book, *Helping Yourself With Foot Reflexology*. I used to be tired all the time. Now hardly ever so. I know it works."

Mrs. A.N. N.

14

How Reflexology Can Cure Your Headache

As an illustration of how pain can be squeezed out of the top of the head through the fingers, a typical case reported by Dr. George Starr White may be helpful.

A lady suffered from a severe headache on the top of her head, which had persisted for more than three weeks. She had consulted several doctors who had given her drugs and hypodermics, but the relief was only temporary.

Doctor White told her nothing of what was contemplated, but took hold of her hands and began firmly pressing on the first, second, and third fingers—the pain being diffused over the frontal regions—at the same time engaging her in conversation concerning her condition. After about three minutes, he asked her if she could indicate with her hand just where the pain was.

She hesitated, looked up, and said, "Do you use mental therapy?" Then, after blinking perplexedly for half a minute, she added, "For the first time in three weeks, except when I've been under the influence of narcotics, the pain is entirely gone." Doctor White told her to have someone repeat these finger pressures, at the same time emphasizing that if she failed to get relief from this method, to come back. He has not seen her since.

Now, remember that the same condition might not be cleared up from the same point every time, even in the same patient. At one time we might stop it by pressing the forefinger, and another time the point would be found some place on the thumb, or maybe the middle finger, or even in the webs. (See Figures 8 and 22 in the front of the book).

HEADACHE FROM OTHER CAUSES

In many cases, headaches can be caused from the eyes and also from the stomach. If the finger massage doesn't stop the head pain in a few minutes, then try the reflexes to the stomach. (See Chart #2). The reflexes to the stomach will be found near the web between the thumb and index finger, and also slightly over into the center of the hand.

Press this with the rolling motion learned earlier in the book. Be careful in massaging this area very long if you have an upset or weak stomach, as it might make you nauseated. Don't let this stop you from massaging the stomach reflexes, however, as this will give you a healthy, strong stomach in time. So keep at it, slowly at first.

You will be amazed at how quickly you will forget that you ever had a stomachache or a headache.

Now, the headache could also be caused from a pinched nerve in the neck or spine. If this is the case, then we would work on the thumb and also the big toe if it is convenient to do so. I have many letters from people all over the world telling me of the wonderful results they received in curing their headaches after following directions in my book on Foot Reflexology.

On the foot, you can roll and rotate the big toe, which will have the neck reflexes, the same as the thumb. Then you can follow right on down the foot on the spine reflexes. But on the hand, you will remember it is a little different.

The reflexes to the back are on the bone leading down the hand in back of the thumb, as shown in Chart #2. (See Figure 5 in the front of the book.)

How Reflexology Helped a Square-Dancer

My husband and I were at a square dance festival a few days ago, when a very good friend came up to tell us good-bye. Since it was early in the evening, we asked why they were leaving before the dance was over. His wife said that he had a terrible headache. I had noticed that he had been quite listless earlier in the evening. My husband showed him how to press the top or back of the thumb, with the thumb of the opposite hand until he found a tender place and then to continue to massage it for a few minutes, or until the headache was better. We thought they had gone home until we saw them later. They were dancing and his eyes looked bright and free from pain. They danced the rest of the evening, even joining the crowd for dinner later. He said he felt completely free from his headache, thanks to the thumb massage, even if it was hard to believe. He told us later that the headaches had been frequent for years but now he knew how to prevent them from starting and was very grateful.

Appreciative People Spread the News of Reflexology

It would indeed be a marvelous sum total of health, happiness, and economic efficiency if all headaches, for instance, would be cured, and kept cured, by Reflexology.

Many appreciative people are spreading the knowledge of this wonderful technique of simply massaging the fingers and toes, and to do away with the need for resorting to dangerous drugs! We must carry this teaching to its only logical conclusion and teach how, by perfectly safe and harmless means, people may, if sick, cure themselves of their minor ailments! If your doctor can't help you, why not try Reflexology? It is safe! And everyone receives some benefit. At one time there were many very prominent physicians, osteopaths, chiropractors, and even dentists who used Reflexology, popularly known as "Zone Therapy," to relieve pain.

How a Hangover was Quickly Relieved

Reflexology will even relieve headache from a hangover. My husband was with a fishing party where some of the men spent one evening drinking. One of the men complained of a terrible headache the next morning. Nothing he took seemed to bring relief. My husband told him to rub his thumb with the opposite thumb and forefinger. He looked skeptical, but being in pain, he tried it, and was amazed that his headache was gone almost instantly. He went around telling everyone about it. And he said he felt great, too—no more hangover!

The next time you have a headache, instead of attempting to paralyze the nerves of sensation with an opiate or pain deadener, try massaging the thumb. You will find it rather tender at first but keep massaging it a few minutes and feel the wonderful relief as the pain lifts from you.

If the headache is in the middle of the head, massaging the

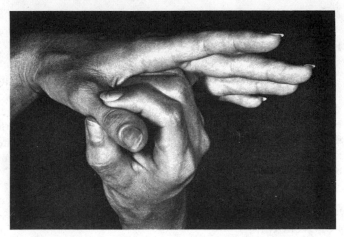

Figure 14-1. Position for massaging reflexes in the thumb.

thumb reflex will usually stop it in a very few minutes, and in many cases almost immediately. (See Figure 14-1.)

If it persists, then massage the finger next to it, also. As I described in my book on Foot Reflexology, massaging the big toe stopped most headaches almost immediately. And I have many letters telling of the success of those who have used this method to stop their headaches with nothing else but massaging their big toes! But in many cases it is easier and more convenient to massage the thumb. This can be done even in public without being noticed by anyone. You will find that it will also relieve nervousness.

Headaches Due to Neck Tension or Eye Weaknesses Relieved

Tension in the neck causes many headaches and eye weaknesses. We have many reports of relief from these complaints when people used this method of massaging the big toe as described in my book on Foot Reflexology.

As you can see on Chart #2, the thumb represents the head and neck. After we have given the thumb a good massage, let us take it between the thumb and first two fingers of the opposite hand and start to roll it first to the right and then to the left, around and around several times each way, and soon you will find yourself relaxing. It gives the same relaxing sensation that you would get if someone took your head in his hands and gently rolled it around and around, from side to side.

15

How to Stimulate the Thyroid Gland with Reflex Massage

Now let's talk about the thyroid reflexes in the hands. Study Charts #2 and #3 in the beginning of this book, and note where the thyroid is located in the body, and also the reflexes to the thyroid in the hands. Now look at Figure 15-1 and note how the reflex to the thyroid is being massaged.

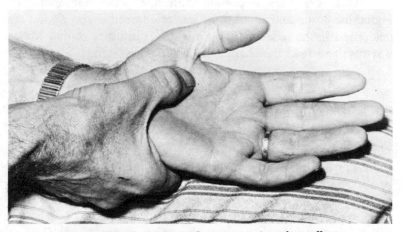

Figure 15-1.   Position for massaging the reflex to the thyroid gland.

Notice how the thumb of the right hand is pressing under the bone of the pad just under the left thumb, inside of the large thumb pad toward the center of the hand.

Start at the base of the thumb bone near the wrist, pressing along this pad. Use a pressing and rolling motion with the thumb of the right hand and follow the inner edge of the pad on up to the web between the thumb and index finger. It may be easier to use a massager on this particular reflex area as shown in Figure 9-2 in the chapter on devices. This is especially true for most men since their hands are inclined to be toughened by hard use through the years.

Using the thumb of the opposite hand, press along this pad until you hit the reflex to the thyroid. If you have any kind of thyroid congestion, you will experience a sharp pain when you press it. The whole area may be quite tender, with the pain quite pronounced at first, but as you continue the massage with the rolling-pressing motion the crystals will be broken loose and washed away by the increased flow of blood. You will notice the pain becoming less and less each time that you massage this area.

Remember, don't get carried away and massage any of these reflexes very long at a time the first few days. You may find that the tenderness is not as sharp and painful in the hands as it is in the feet due to the daily use of the hands, in comparison with the protection of our feet by shoes, soft carpets, sidewalks, and lawns to walk on.

This is a very important hormone producing gland of the endocrine group and is not to be neglected even if you do not feel the tenderness in the reflex that you might feel in other glands. Massage it anyway, and read the chapter on Endocrine Glands.

REFLEXES TO THE PARATHYROID GLANDS

If you will study Chart #3 of the Endocrine Glands, you will notice the location of the tiny parathyroid glands. As you can see, there are two on each side of the thyroid and they lie just in back of the lobes. You can easily see that you will use the same location and the same massage for these very important tiny glands. You will have to press a little deeper to reach them. Massaging for these in the feet is more simple than massaging them in the hands. You would almost have to use some type of massager, such as the Hand Massager as shown in Figure 9-2 and Figure 1 in the front of the book, or the Magic Reflex Massager will also work here. If you do not have these, you can use a pencil with an eraser which will serve you quite well. Since they are so small, you will have to use your own judgment in massaging them. The parathyroids will generally get enough stimulation when you massage the reflexes to the thyroid, unless there is a definite congestion within them.

The thyroid and parathyroids are responsible for your poise and tranquility and well-being, besides many other important body functions which I will describe in another chapter.

Although you will not be so apt to bruise the tissues or capillaries in the hands with the deep massage as you would in the feet, nevertheless, be discreet in how hard you press, especially if you are using some device with which to massage.

In massaging the reflexes in the hands, we also use compression massage on the fingers with added help. As I said before, the hands, unlike the feet, do not have much room for all the reflexes of the body, thus we also find that we get added benefits by stimulating the reflexes in the fingers.

If you do not have my book, "Helping Yourself With Foot Reflexology," the thyroid reflexes on the feet would be just under the pad of the big toe, the same as under the pad of the thumb. Be sure to massage this reflex in both hands and if you massage the foot reflexes, do it on both feet. Never leave half of the body untreated.

Reflexology Helps Friends in the Caribbean Islands

Dear Mrs. Carter:

Just a few lines to let you know that receiving your book on "Reflexology" was the answer to my prayers.

I am a man 65 years old and I was suffering with pains and aches all over. Ever since I applied reflexology, I feel like a new man. Thanks to you. I have been treating friends of mine and I have recommended your book, if they want to follow their treatments.

During my vacation, I went to the Caribbean Islands. In Puerto Rico, I met a man who told me that two of the fingers of his left hand were numb. He was afraid to wear his expensive rings for fear that they might drop off and he would not know about it. I gave him a treatment and to his surprise and mine his fingers were O.K.

In the Dominican Republic, we visited a family of friends,

and met a lady who was suffering from pains all over the right side of the head, neck and shoulder. She said "Sometimes the pain goes down to the leg." I offered to give her right side a treatment which she accepted. We went away and when we returned three hours later we stopped to inquire if the treatment had done anything for her and the answer I got was that she grabbed me, hugged and kissed me.

To tell you the truth Mrs. Carter, they made me feel like a big shot. One drawback is the senoritas thought that I was the man they had been waiting for and proposed marriage to me.

Well, Mrs. Carter, may the Good Lord bless you and I beg to remain your healthful friend.

C.G.

16

How to Massage for Lung and Respiratory Problems

Let us look at Chart #2 and see the position of the lungs; notice how they lie in the chest and then notice how the reflexes to the lungs are situated along the pad under the fingers, just below the eye and ear reflexes. You will also notice that the lungs take quite a large space in the chest area; similarly, the reflexes to the lungs take up quite an area on the hand. Remember, right lung, right hand; left lung, left hand.

For position to massage the lungs, take the left hand in the right hand, using the thumb to massage along the reflexes on the pad under the fingers; use a walking-pressing motion as you massage this whole reflex area. If you have one defective lung, then you will concentrate on the reflexes of the hand that is on the same side as the affected lung. But don't neglect massaging the other hand completely, also.

If your fingers are not strong, you can use the eraser end on a pencil or use the hand massager if you have one.

Imbalance of Body Caused by Faulty Lungs

Anyone who has any malfunctioning of the lungs naturally has some imbalance in other parts of the body also. If one gland or organ is out of function, then it throws the whole off balance and we end up with a body which is out of harmony with the cosmic vibrations of the universe. So we can see that for any malfunction, no matter how small, we must treat the whole body to put all the instruments back in tune to get perfect harmony.

This is the reason Reflexology seems to be such a miraculous way to health. We don't treat just one malfunctioning part.

HOW REFLEXOLOGY SPEEDS UP HEALING PROCESS

When we press on all of the reflex buttons, we are charging the whole body with a vibrating force of electric energy which stimulates nature into a speeded-up process of healing.

So you can see why you will always give yourself a complete treatment at least every other day while trying to stimulate one certain area that is in malfunction from congestion of one kind or another. This is where the magic of the little Magic Massager comes in. It can press and stimulate most of the reflex buttons in the hand at one time, not only to the lungs but to most of the organs and glands in the body.

If you are treating the lungs you can use the Magic Reflex Massager once or twice a day on both hands. (Never take a half treatment.) Hold it in one hand while you squeeze and roll it around and around, pressing the little fingers into every reflex button in your hand. Now do the same with the other hand. You must not use it over two or three minutes at a time for the first two weeks. Rubber bands, or the reflex clamps placed on all of the fingers on the same side where the offending lung is located, will also be of great help in anesthetizing and healing the offending organ.

IMPORTANCE OF RESPIRATORY SYSTEM

The respiratory system is more important to the perfect functioning of our whole body than most people realize.

The trachea (windpipe) and lungs are parts of the respiratory system, which delivers oxygen to the blood; the blood delivers purified oxygen to the cells of which our bodies are built. Your lungs consist of millions of elastic membrane sacs which together can hold about as much air as a basketball. Do you breathe in that much air, enough air to keep your lungs full? The lungs are constantly inflating and emptying in their crucial capacity as a medium of exchange.

Your lungs sustain your life by unloading carbon dioxide and taking in oxygen carried by the blood to the cells. OXYGEN unlocks the energy contained in your body's fuels. Do you know that your body's trillions of cells require so much OXYGEN that you need about 30 times as much surface for its intake as your entire skin area covers? Your lungs provide this surface area even though they weigh only about 2½ pounds. During moderate activity all the blood in your body passes through your lungs more than 100 times an hour.

Can you see now why your lungs are really the most important organ in your body? You could live several days without water, and several weeks without food, but you cannot live even several minutes without air. It is the "AIR OF LIFE" that nourishes the nucleus of all atoms of all organs in the body.

This air, at all times present and perpetual, is the Creative Substance of all matter! This takes us back to Anaximenes (6th century B.C.) who said; "The essence of the Universe is in the Infinite Air in eternal movement which contains ALL in itself."

When you were born you breathed in THE BREATH OF LIFE immediately or you wouldn't be here today. Are you now beginning to understand the importance of a healthy respiratory system?

17

How Reflexology Can
Help Your Back

The importance of the spine to our general health is familiar to all practitioners. The chiropractic, naturopath, and osteopathic doctors know that the greater part of one's well-being depends on the condition of the spine. To massage the reflexes of the back or spine is to relax the muscle tension surrounding any vertebra that is not in perfect and healthful alignment. Remember that the body can never be in perfect health if the spine is out of alignment.

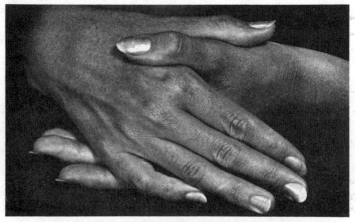

Figure 17.1   Position for pressing reflexes to the back.

You have studied the position of the spine and its reflexes in the hands in Chart #2. Look at Figure 17-1 on massaging the spine reflexes. Notice how the thumb of the left hand is clasped around the center of the right hand. This is where part of the reflexes to the spine are located in the hands.

HOW TO MASSAGE REFLEXES TO THE SPINE

Now, unlike the spine reflex in the foot, following in one straight line from the big toe down, you will look to the index finger as well as the thumb in massaging the neck and the spine.

Take the index finger and feel just at the base of it, finding the reflex first to the vertebra of the spine. Remember that the index finger and also the thumb represent the head and the neck of your body. Notice how this bone represents the spine as it goes in a straight line from the index finger, clear down to the base of the thumb at the wrist, ending just in back of the thumb, which would

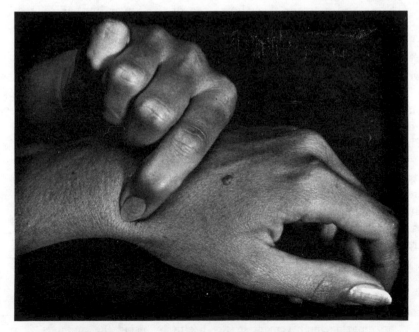

Figure 17-2. A position for massaging reflexes to the coccyx (end of spine).

be the reflexes to the lower back area. Notice in Figure 17-2, how the thumb is pressing into the lower back reflex area or lower lumbar region.

If you have lower back trouble, then you should look for tenderness in this area. If you have back ache in the center of the back, then look for tenderness in the center of the hand, as in Figure 17-3. If there is pain or tension in the upper part of the back, as between the shoulders or neck, look for tenderness just below the index finger, then follow this bony structure down to the wrist (Figure 5 in the front of the book).

Using the pressing, rolling motion, as you work your way down this ridge, search out the tender spots with the fingers and massage them a few seconds as you find them remembering that neck reflexes are also in the thumb.

In some of these tender places you may find it more beneficial just to hold with a steady pressure for a few seconds, especially in the reflexes to the spine. You will soon learn what seems to be the best for your particular case.

Press and massage the whole area of the lower lumbar reflexes (See Figure 17-4 for lumbar and coccyx), using the thumb and the fingers with a pressing and rolling motion all the way around the wrist. Yes, the front and the back of the wrist and the outside of the wrist also.

Notice when you are pressing on the lower lumbar reflex on the thumb side, that just on the other side of the thumb, on the palm side of the hand, that you are very near to the bladder reflex. See Chart #2.

Note on the chart that the whole spinal column is located in the exact center of the body. In the foot, the reflexes cover the entire area of the inside of each foot, lengthwise from the toe to the heel. But in the hands we do not have as much of an area for the reflexes as we do in the feet, so they have to be placed in a more congested area.

Injured Back Helped by Reflexology

Mr. M. reports:

I received your book on Reflexology and have brought about an amazing improvement in my health by using the methods put forth by Mrs. Carter.

I injured my back several years ago and after using these

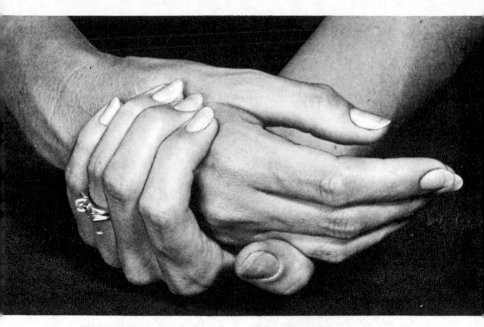

Figure 17-3. Position for massaging the reflexes to the spine.

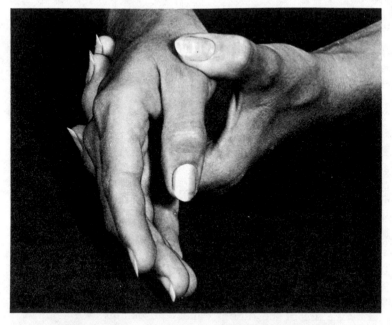

Figure 17-4. Position for massaging the reflexes to the lower back and coccyx.

methods I have been free of pain for the first time in years. I sleep like a baby and feel years younger. I have treated some of my friends, bringing relief from sinus congestion, sore throats, muscular pains, and so forth.

I can't thank Mrs. Carter and you the publisher enough for putting these wonderful health secrets in print.

Many Causes of Backache

A few years ago, all back trouble was called lumbago. We know now that there are many causes of backache. Besides the vertebra being out of alignment or a slipped disc, etc., backache can be caused by malfunctioning kidneys, lack of calcium, female disorders. arthritis, and other causes.

Doctor Bowers claims that Zone Therapy (Reflexology) is one of the most valuable methods for treating obstinate conditions. He states, "Lumbago, as a rule, responds very quickly to Zone Therapy. Cases who come to the office 'all doubled up' are straightened out, frequently in one treatment, and wend their way homeward rejoicing."

Comb to Ease Back Pain

Another successful method of treating back troubles is the use of the reflex comb. (See Figure 6-2 in Chapter 6.) It is a metal-type comb with dull pointed teeth and a spur on the end to use as pressure in the thumb region when using pressure massage on the hands. From the position of massaging the web, roll the comb till the teeth press into the spine reflexes, and massage.

The teeth are pressed firmly into the palms of the hands, and on the palm side of the thumb. Also press the teeth of the comb into the ends of the first, second, and third fingers. For best results, you should continue this pressure for about ten to twenty minutes. If one side of the back is in pain, work on the hand on the same side. You may also work on the web between the thumb and the first and second fingers as explained in Chapter 6.

In my private practice I had wonderful results simply by massaging the reflexes in the feet. Dr. Bowers cites some very amazing results from this comb method of treatment, to relieve backache— and also by the use of the rubber bands and clamps as explained in Chapter 8. For many of you, this will be an easier method than trying to reach the feet.

How Reflexology Relieves Minister of Back Pains

A minister who for weeks, had been unable to turn in bed without assistance was, after a twenty-minute treatment, able to arise and walk unaided. He was entirely relieved of pain and discomfort within a few hours, and the next day he was "up and around."

Relief almost always follows the first treatment, apparently regardless of the cause of the back trouble.

Man Cured of Back Pain in a Few Minutes

Dr. Bowers tells of a case of backache which had persisted for more than three months. This gentleman had taken practically every form of treatment that could be recommended by the most able specialists; he had even been to Hot Springs. He was bent almost double, and for many weeks had not been able to stand erect. He was given two metal combs and told to squeeze them for ten or fifteen minutes, while waiting in the anteroom. After he was brought into the office, his hands were thoroughly "combed" by pressure, from finger tip to wrist. He straightened out completely after this first treatment, and expressed himself as entirely relieved from pain. He received a similar treatment the following day, after which he went his way rejoicing.

"These results are practically uniform. I know of many scores of patients thus cured with a comb," states Dr. Bowers.

The clothespin method, explained in another chapter, and also the rubber band method are sometimes used with equally good results.

Train Conductor Relieved of Back Pain

One doctor, a reflex massage enthusiast, while on a trip to a Shriners' convention, noticed that the conductor of the train walked "all doubled up" and seemed to be suffering great pain. It developed that the railroad man had a "misery in his back," had given up work, and gone to a sanitarium for three weeks—without obtaining much relief. Three days prior to his resuming work he had not been able to straighten up or make any sudden move without suffering excruciatingly.

He was invited to come to the smoking compartment for a few minutes, where the doctor put rubber bands on the thumb and forefingers of both the trainman's hands, and at the same time made firm pressure with his thumb nails on these same fingers. The conductor was not informed of the purpose of this procedure, so his imagination had nothing to work on.

After holding his fingers in this manner for about ten minutes, the whistle blew and the conductor had to leave his chair suddenly. He straightened up and went out on the run. When he came back he laughed and said, "This is the first time in six weeks I've gotten up or moved without pain. What in thunder have those little rubber bands got to do with lumbago, anyway?"

The doctor saw the man before leaving the train two hours later, and he was still free from pain.

These results can be duplicated by anyone who will apply the simple techniques outlined in this book.

There are so many natural methods to alleviate suffering and disease that I could go on forever telling you of them.

Reflexology Saves Man from Operation
on Spine

One case I had was a man in his thirties, with a back so bad that he was unable to do any manual labor of any kind. I have been in his home when he turned to say "good-by," and went crashing to the floor. He had to crawl to a chair to help himself slowly up. The doctors told him he had a slipped disc and he would only get worse, as the disc was deteriorating and could not possibly get better. They claimed an operation was imperative. I talked him into letting me give him some reflex treatments to see what reflexology could do for him. In a very short time, Mr. B. was free from all back trouble. He was able to do all kinds of manual work, such as roofing his house, hiking, etc. That was 17 years ago and he still has a good strong back. I wonder how he would be, if he had undergone an operation?

18

How Reflexology Can Help Your Heart

Heart disease, including certain circulatory disorders, is on the increase, and results in more deaths than do the next four or five diseases combined. Not only does it strike those who are in an advanced age, but it is a threat to many in the prime of life. It is even one of the chief threats to life and health among college students of today. We are no longer surprised to hear of a young child who has collapsed and died from heart failure.

WHAT THE HEART IS AND HOW IT WORKS

The heart is a muscular organ with walls ranging from one-quarter to three-quarters of an inch in thickness. It is actually a pump which circulates the blood throughout the body. In the blood itself are the red corpuscles that take up and discharge oxygen during circulation. The whole process is continuous and takes about a minute for the blood to make a complete double circle through the body. Do you know that this heart muscle actually takes a rest after each beat longer than the beat itself?

You can see, as you study Chart #2, that the heart is located on the left side of the body, a part of it extending over into the center.

Notice in Figure 18-1 how the thumb of the right hand is pressed into the pad under the little finger. Remember that since the heart and its circulatory system extend over into the center of the

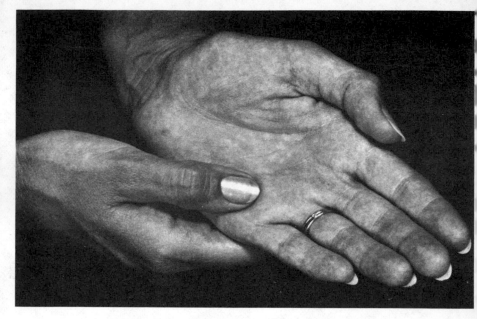

Figure 18-1. Massaging the reflexes to the heart.

body, you will press and massage this whole area, working the thumb clear over into the reflexes to the stomach and webs, searching for tender spots as you go. When the sore spots are found, work them out, as they are telling you of congestion in this particular place. See Figure 7 in the front of this book.

By looking at Charts #1 and #2, we will see how the meridian Zone Lines Number 1 through 5 run through the area of the heart from the first to the fifth fingers, so you know that by holding pressure on these fingers you will be calming the heart. When you use massage on this heart reflex area, you are activating the vital life force into the canals to help nature relieve congestion and revive glandular activity.

How Heart Pain Can be Relieved with Reflexology

The heart can be aided with the reflex push buttons, no matter what the nature of the trouble is. I have treated heart complaints many times while we waited for the doctor to arrive, or until I was sure the afflicted one was out of danger and free from pain.

If there is pain in the chest or heart region, then the reflexes to the whole area should be massaged. If there are pains going along the arm and shoulder, which is characteristic of angina pectoris, then you will work the whole region, even up onto the little finger and the one next to it. Here we are trying to relieve tension. You may also use clamps on all of the fingers of the left hand.

Many cases of death have been laid to heart failure, when the underlying causes are actually the poor condition of other glands which puts so much overwork on the heart that it finally gives up.

People put an extra load on the heart by filling the lungs with nicotine and polluted air. They fail to eat the proper foods, yet wonder why they are stricken with a heart attack just when they were getting ready to enjoy life, not realizing that congestion has been accumulating for years in the veins around the heart and other organs.

How a Signal Forewarns of Heart Attack

While visiting my parents, I talked with their neighbor, Mr. D., a middle-aged man who had a history of heart attacks and was a semi-invalid. I said to him one day, "If I tell you where to rub your feet for your heart, will you do it?" He looked at me rather oddly and said, "Oh, I suppose I would do anything if I thought it would help." I knew how doubtful he felt. "Can you reach your feet with your hands?" I asked. "Yes, I can still do that," he replied. So I told him, "You rub all around your little toe on the left foot, massaging especially on the pad just below the toe. Also do the same thing on the little finger of the left hand, and you may not have any more heart attacks."

Suddenly, his head came up and he really looked interested. "Why," he said in a surprised voice, "you know every time before I have an attack I noticed my little toe turns blue. I wondered about this, even mentioned it to my doctor, but no one knew the answer."

He said it started to turn blue several days before the attack. I told him, "If you had massaged it, maybe you would have prevented the attack." "I bet you are right," he said. "I will sure work on my little toe and fingers from now on."

Nature's Barometer May Warn of Heart Weakness

Can this be nature's warning signal telling us that the heart is in need of help? I suggest watching this little barometer carefully if

you are troubled with a heart condition. Massage all the reflexes to
the heart as directed in the preceding pages. The Magic Massager
would also be useful here since it stimulates most of the glands in
the whole body. As you squeeze and roll it in the hands, press the
little fingers into all of the reflex buttons. Be sure to massage the
reflexes in both hands every time as the whole body may be out of
harmony and you are merely helping nature put it back in tune by
massaging all of the reflexes and giving her a chance to bring new
life to the congested glands and dying cells in your body. Yes, health
can be quickly and simply restored through reflexology.

How a Business Man Prevents Heart Attack

Mr. S. told me about an experience he had not long ago in
his office. "While I was working at my desk," he said, "I
suddenly began to feel funny. My chest began to tighten up, I
became nauseated, and pain started to travel up my left arm.
I knew the signs of a heart attack as I had had one several years
ago. As you know, I am an old reflexology enthusiast so I knew
what to do. I just relaxed back in my chair without anyone
noticing and started to massage the pad under my little finger
on my left hand with the thumb of my right hand. I massaged
clear across the hand to the reflexes near the web. I found the
tender spot close to the stomach reflex and massaged it until
it was no longer sore. I kept working on all of the heart reflexes
for about a half hour even though the pain had begun to subside as soon as I started to massage the reflexes in my hand.
No one in the office was aware that anything was wrong and
I was able to resume work in a normal manner, which I am sure
would not have been possible had I not known the value of
reflex massage. I have never had any trouble since, and I know
I never will so long as I use the magic of reflex massage."

Let me give you a word of warning while we are on the subject
of the heart. *Don't overdo!* Never overdo! Remember that your heart
is a muscle and when your outer muscles become flabby, so do your
inner muscles, like your heart. If your legs and arms are very soft
from lying around idle for a long time, you wouldn't try to go out
and run a foot race or play a game of tennis or ball just because you
felt good one day, would you? If you did, you would probably have
muscle spasms in your arms and legs.

The heart is a muscle, too, a big muscle in proportion to the size of the body. In the male, the heart weighs from 10 to 12 ounces. If you overtaxed it with unusual exercise before giving it a chance to build up strength after a long rest, it could very easily have a muscle spasm, too—heart attack! This is what often happens when men walk out of an office where they spend most of their time sitting and go on a hunting trip, for instance.

Let me give you an example in the experience of Mr. B.

Man Recovers Too Quickly

Mr. B. came to me after suffering for months from a heart condition. He took about three treatments from me in a period of seven days and felt so well he decided to go back to work. He was sure he was well. I tried to tell him his heart was still soft from his months of inactivity. I told him, "Give your heart a chance to build up its strength. Wait awhile, give your heart a chance." He felt so good he wouldn't listen and drove over one hundred miles to ask for his old job back. He felt like a new man. He walked all over the factory and up and down many flights of stairs. He then walked up a long hill to his parked car. This is when his heart began to protest. After that, he went back into semi-invalidism.

He never came back to me. He had lost faith in this great work that might have made him a healthy man for the rest of his life if he had only listened, or used common sense.

So, remember Mr. B., and no matter how well you feel after massaging your reflexes, give your body time to build up strength and muscle and you will feel like a new man all your life.

How Dr. Shute Cures Heart Patients

Of course, we all know of the wonderful results Doctor Wilfrid E. Shute of Shute Foundation, London, Canada has obtained with heart patients by using Vitamin E in his hospital. This, combined with reflex massage, and vitamins, should put the rate of death from heart disease down to the bottom of the list.

19

How to Use Reflex Massage for a Stroke

If you have had a stroke or are in danger of having one, reflexology can be your salvation. Since the reflexes to the head are located mainly in the area of the thumb, you will massage all parts of the thumb with the thumb and finger of the opposite hand. You press and roll all parts of the thumb, concentrating on the back under the thumb nail, also the sides. You are searching for a tender spot if you have had a stroke and finding it, you will then concentrate on massaging it. You will also massage all of the thumb.

When you find an extremely tender spot in the thumb, it is indicative of the reflex to the brain damage caused by the stroke. You should also massage the next two fingers near the thumb, and always massage the web as explained in Chapter 6. If the damage is more to the side of the head, then you may have to go to the fourth and fifth fingers, massaging fingers on both hands but concentrating, of course, on the side on which the stroke damage is located. Pressure by reflex clamps, rubber bands or other devices may be used as explained in the chapter 8. See Figure 14 in the front of the book.

A comb can also be used to good advantage to exert pressure on these reflexes, holding the pressure from five to twenty minutes.

Massage for High Blood Pressure to Prevent Stroke

Since high blood pressure is connected with strokes, you will want to concentrate on the reflexes to the liver on the right hand (see Figure 20-1 in the next chapter), and also on the reflexes to the pituitary gland which are located in the thumbs as shown on Chart #2 and Figure 5-1 in Chapter 5.

We can see that since a stroke is caused by some malfunction of the body, why it is so important to treat all of the reflexes to help stimulate the flow of the life force to every gland and organ, thus helping nature restore the whole body back to its natural balance and harmony with the universe.

Remember, when one instrument is out of tune it causes the whole orchestra to be out of harmony, and, like a great orchestra, when one of your glands is malfunctioning your health goes into a rasping discord.

So, never neglect massaging all of the reflexes at least two times a week when you are treating a certain illness or just for general health reasons.

Although I helped many people recover from strokes when I had an office, I would like to include here reports from others who have had success with this method of treatment after using the directions as given in my former book on Foot Reflexology. However, the treatment is as effective with hand reflex massage, in most cases.

Stroke Victim Helped by Reflexology

Mr. A. reports. "My wife had a stroke several years ago but her progress was very slow and doctors didn't seem to do anything about it. About six weeks ago I purchased your book on Foot Reflexology, and started to give my wife treatments. To our surprise, it worked miracles, and in this short time she is almost back to normal and still improving. The doctors are dumbfounded and can't figure it out. I haven't told them, as they would only ridicule it."

How a Brain-Damaged Victim Recovers

Mrs. H. gives the following report. "I am more convinced then ever that reflexology really works. I just finished a case where I had an occasion to use this type of therapy.

"My patient was a cardiac arrest and was comatose for three days. She also had brain damage which affected her equilibrium. The doctors said she would not walk for at least six months, if ever. She had uremic poisoning and other complications. The doctor told me I could give her the massage. The first week I gave her two treatments, and the very second day I observed an almost immediate response. Within three weeks, she was walking with help, and in one month she was walking alone and was discharged from the hospital. I went home with her and continued treating her for two weeks, twice a week. She is now as good as she ever was and is out working in her garden every day."

20

How to Use Reflexes
to Help the Liver

The liver is the largest body organ. It is also the most versatile. It is estimated that the liver has, roughly, five hundred jobs to do. You can see the importance of giving this busy organ all the help it needs. Among other functions, it receives about one-fourth of the arterial blood pumped out by the heart at every beat, and all the blood from the veins in the area of the intestines which contain digested food; it removes toxic substances such as nicotine, alcohol, caffeine, drugs, industrial poisons, etc. from the blood, and acts on foodstuff already reduced by the digestive process by putting it back together in chemical compounds usable by the body.

The liver has been called "the main factory and storehouse" of the body. It manufactures and secretes bile, necessary for digestion, and stores it in the gall bladder which releases it into the duodenum, as if on signal as soon as the stomach has passed it along, when the food you eat starts on its journey on its complicated course to keep your body nourished and functioning. The liver stores vitamins and releases them as required by the body, as well as glycogen which it restores to the bloodstream as glucose when needed. As a blood purifier, it removes such waste products as worn out red blood cells and hormones in excess of the body's needs, in addition to toxic substances. It not only manufactures coagulants which keep you from bleeding to death but also anticoagulants that keep your blood from thickening dangerously in the arteries.

Because of this heavy load imposed on it, the liver is distensible.

This interesting and indispensable organ has the power to rebuild itself if given a chance even after a large part of it has been destroyed by disease.

It is not possible to go into great detail about the liver's numerous functions but you can see that this important health-builder needs all the stimulation it can get in order to keep the body functioning in perfect order.

TECHNIQUE OF MASSAGING THE LIVER REFLEXES

As you can see from Chart #2, the reflexes to the liver are rather crowded within a comparatively small area of the hand. Study the chart for the exact location.

You will use the thumb of the left hand to massage the reflexes on the right hand. Remember that the liver is on the right side of the body, so the reflex to it is on the right hand.

Use the side or tip of the left thumb and press with the rolling motion, starting just under the little finger. Massage this area firmly, checking for a tender spot that might give you a warning signal that the liver has become sluggish and needs your life-giving help by sending renewed vitality and life force to this important organ.

Don't be afraid to massage a large area here, remembering that the liver is the largest organ in the body and the reflexes will be found in a larger area of the hand.

Finger-Squeezing for the Liver

You may also find that there will be tender spots in the web between the thumb and index finger of the right hand when the liver is malfunctioning. As stated previously, the webs between the fingers seem to be a special center for reflexes to several parts of the body so don't neglect to massage these when giving yourself a treatment.

After pressing the webs between the fingers checking for sore spots, we will learn how to squeeze certain fingers which will not only work as an anesthetic if there is pain, but will help in the healing process as well. Let us move up to the first joint of the three outside fingers, which will be #3, #4, and #5 as shown on Chart #1. Press these fingers with the fingers of the left hand, first from the sides, and then the front and back of each finger.

Rubber bands or Reflex Clamps may be applied for a few

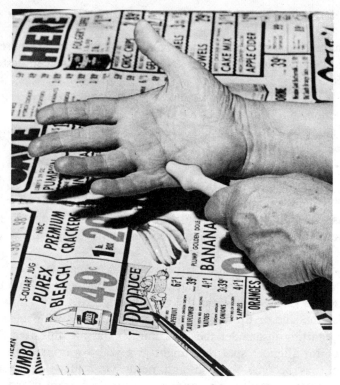

Figure 20-1. Massaging the reflexes to the liver with hand massager before a shopping trip.

minutes to give a steady pressure on these reflexes which will not only act to deaden pain but also to stimulate the electric life force of nature to heal the areas to which these reflexes are connected. You may also use the Hand Massager shown in Figure 20-1.

Use of the Comb for Liver Reflex Massage

You can use the comb technique in massaging reflexes to the liver as well as many other glands, as explained in Chapter 8.

Taking the comb in the right hand and pressing the ends of the three outer fingers on the teeth of the comb will help stimulate the liver into new life. You may also press the comb into the reflex to the liver on the right hand by turning the comb over with the teeth down, and using fingers to apply pressure, for an extra stimulus.

Traveler Uses Steering Wheel to Relieve Liver Complaints

Mrs. L.C.P. reports, "I woke up this morning with a dull ache in the region of my liver and gall bladder, accompanied by a headache, both of which I attributed to having over-eaten a lot of rich foods at a late dinner party last night. I had an early appointment some ten miles from home, and I wondered if it were safe to drive that far. I decided to risk it, and as I drove the car, I massaged both hands vigorously by rotating them on the steering wheel with a rather firm grip. Both the headache and the pain disappeared in a matter of minutes and did not return, allowing me to go about my business."

Stomach and Gall Bladder Relieved

Dear Mildred Carter:

I am studying this book "Helping Yourself with Foot Reflexology" and I just want to tell you how beneficial I am finding the instructions. Pains in the stomach and over the gall bladder were relieved almost at once.

Thank you,
Very truly,
M.F., Florida

21

How Reflex Massage Can Help Your Stomach

Everyone knows what it is to have a stomachache. The stomach is the most abused part of your whole body. It has to take care of everything that is pushed into it through the mouth, and very few people care what they feed into this loyal hard-working servant, or how they present it. Yet, it strives to accept and separate and dispose of each separate parcel into the right channels after it receives it, besides all the unhealthy, indigestible liquids containing alcohol, sugar, harmful additives and acids which also have to be separated into their proper disposal channels. Food was intended to be chewed by man until it was acted upon by the saliva in the mouth. Do you take time to chew your food to liquid before you swallow it? If you do, you probably are enjoying perfect health today and have no need for trying to find a way back to health.

The entry of food into the stomach—as well as its exit—is regulated by circular muscles which act somewhat like purse strings, alternately expanding and contracting. The stomach works on the food both mechanically and chemically. The movement of the stomach mashes the food, kneading it as a cook kneads dough. This permits the thorough mixing in of digestive juices, the main ones being pepsin and hydrochloric acid.

You will see in Diagram #1 in the next chapter how the stomach and its related organs work. This will give you some idea of what goes on in various parts of the ailmentary canal. With the help of this diagram, you can follow the long journey which food makes through the food canal of your body.

HOW THE STOMACH TAKES CARE OF FOOD

There are three different kinds of juices released by the salivary glands in the mouth which must be mixed with the food as it is chewed and before it passes down the ten-inches-long gullet into the stomach. These glands are located as follows: one under the tongue, one near the hinge of the jaw and one near the inner ear.

While the food is in the stomach, gastric juices, produced at the rate of over six pints a day, soften it to the consistency of a paste. From time to time, a valve opens and allows small quantities of this paste to pass to the curving tube of the duodenum. Two small pipes lead into the duodenum, one from the liver and another from the pancreas.

Can you now see why those persons who are victims of a duodenal ulcer have such a difficult time healing it?

In Diagram #1 you will notice that the stomach lies to the left, whereas in the chart you see the stomach illustrated in the center of the body. As I have said before, the charts are not drawn to scale, but merely to help you find the correct locations of the reflexes responding to them. See Figure 2 in front of book.

Now that you understand a little of the complicated work the stomach has to do, you can easily see how it needs all the cooperation it can get. Let us begin sending the healing forces of nature to activate this all-important organ with the electric energy of the life forces of the universe by stimulating the reflexes to the stomach and its related parts.

MASSAGING TECHNIQUE TO RELIEVE
STOMACH TROUBLES

Since the stomach is located more to the left side, let us start with the reflexes on the left hand. If you will look at Figure 21-1, you will see how the thumb of the right hand is pressing into the soft spongy area of the left hand near the pad of the thumb and near the web. You will massage this area with a rolling pressing motion for a few minutes. If you start to feel nauseated, stop; leave it alone for a few minutes, then massage the same area on the right hand as shown. Although the stomach lies mostly on the left side, it is affected by the same reflexes in both hands as the duodenum and the pancreas extend over to the right side.

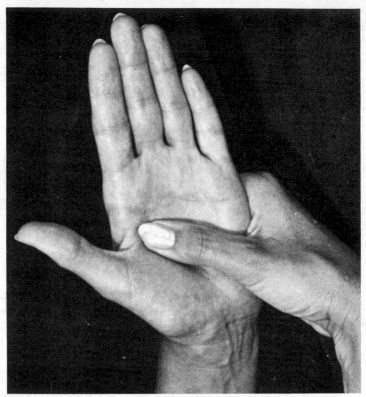

Figure 21-1. Position for massaging the reflexes to the stomach and the colon.

Now turn to massaging the web between the thumb and first finger as this seems to have a very intimate connection with the stomach. If you are using the clamps or bands, place them on fingers 1, 2 3 and 4; thus, you will also be stimulating the salivary glands in the area of the head, plus other glands and organs which could be the cause of your stomach trouble.

Different Ways to Help Your Stomach with Reflexology

The metal reflex comb may be used by pressing the teeth into the different reflexes of the stomach. Now that you know the importance your stomach plays in your well being, you will want to find the method that seems to work best for you, or you may use all of them. Search for tender spots in these areas and when you find them, *work them out.*

Combing the Reflexes to Quiet a Sick Stomach

Another way you may use the comb to quiet a sick stomach is by scratching the back of the hand, using the teeth of the comb. We call this "combing" the reflexes. You just comb the back of the hands, starting at the fingers, and combing down onto the wrists. Don't use any pressure, just the weight of the comb. If you do not have a comb handy, you may use the fingernails instead with a light scratching motion.

How Reflexology Freed Travelers from Carsickness

A friend of mine flew out from the East Coast with her father. When we talked of showing her the beautiful scenery of Oregon, she refused, informing us that riding made her carsick. Her father wanted to go to the coast by car. She was afraid to go, knowing the roads were quite winding most of the way. I asked her if she would take a chance on giving reflexology a try. She agreed to try it as she loves the ocean and wanted very badly to see the Pacific.

We experimented and found that by rubbing the little fingers and the ones next to them, (in the ear reflex area) all signs of carsickness ceased. She was able to travel every place from that day on with no more fear of being sick every time she got into a car. She and her father had a wonderful time sight-seeing the rest of the time she was here.

If you have a like problem of car sickness from riding or any other reason, try massaging these fingers and the ear area for relief. Also massage the webs between the fingers. If it works for others, it can work for you.

How to Stop Baby's Crying with Reflexology

This method may be used to quiet the baby when he is crying at the top of his voice. If a few minutes of combing his hands does not stop the crying, then try gentle pressure on the stomach reflexes, and also on the backs of the hands.

Reflexology Helps Many Stomach Complaints

Reflex massage is valuable in indigestion, nausea, vomiting and all forms of stomach disorders. It has also been used successfully in cases of gastric ulcer. Morning sickness from pregnancy is also helped by the use of this method of massaging the reflexes to the stomach.

How Reflexology Can Stop Carsickness and Seasickness

Carsickness and seasickness can be overcome with reflexology as well as other types of upset of the stomach. I have been telling you to use the thumb and first and second fingers in most cases in treating the stomach, and you will, of course, continue to use them; but in the case of carsickness, we learn that it is caused mainly from a gland in the inner ear. By looking at Chart #1, you will see that this is in zones four and five, and working on the fourth and fifth fingers will stimulate this area.

I suggest you experiment a little here and find the method which best suits your specific condition. Give each method a chance for ten minutes before going on to another, remembering the web is all-important in the reflexes to the stomach. I have even held the ends of my fingers between my teeth when there was nothing better to hold pressure on several fingers at a time.

I do not recommend the Magic Massager in seasick cases as it stimulates all the internal organs. In seasickness, we want to soothe the stomach, not stimulate it. Rubber bands, the comb, or the clamps may be used for this purpose.

Help for Hiccoughs with Reflex Massage

Many devious ways have been used to end the annoyance of hiccoughing, which in some cases has become quite serious, even to sending the victim to the hospital.

We massage the thumb and next two fingers which are in the same zone as the stomach and the diaphragm. Give special attention to the webs between the thumb and first finger and also the webs next to it. If you still have no relief, then use the tongue-pulling method.

Grasp the tongue between the fingers, as explained in other chapters, and pull it out as far as possible and hold it there. In this way, you cure the spasmodic contraction of the diaphragm (the cause of hiccoughs) by influencing the zone in which the trouble originated.

Doctors Tell of Ulcer Cures with Reflexology

Dr. Reid Kellogg has cured many cases of ulcers in one to ten treatments and others in two or three months, such as those with dangerous hemorrhages and other distressing symptoms. Dr. Kellogg used pressures on the thumb, first, and second fingers of both hands with the comb, and also pressed down on the back of the tongue with a probe.

Dr. Bowers tells us, "In less than a dozen treatments, many patients were able to retain food, and practically conduct the entire subsequent course of their own cure." He further states, "I want to emphasize that these cases were most grave, and that they had received skilled medical attention for many weeks without apparent benefit."

M.D. Stops Stomach Pain In Five Minutes

Dr. Charles R. Clapp, M.D., Los Angeles, tells us of Mrs. R., aged 25, who had pain in the epigastric region for three days, using several remedies without any relief. "I treated the thumb and index finger of the right hand with no result. When I began on the thumb of the left hand, she said with a smile, 'There, that strikes the spot.' In less than five minutes, she was free from pain and has had no return of same. This is another clincher for attacking the correct zone (reflex)."

The stomach is the central point for the nerves and should be given consideration in all cases of nervousness and nervous prostration.

A report was given by Orin W. Joslin, M.D., Medical Director of Dodgeville General Hospital and Pine Grove Sanatorium, Dodgeville, Wisconsin.

January 5, 1918

We have been using Zone Therapy (reflexology) as a routine measure in our hospital and sanatorium, especially for pain, and we very seldom fail to get satisfactory results. We hardly ever think of using morphine any more. We have never had a case of gas pains that did not respond inside of ten minutes to zone therapy (reflexology).

I am sorry that I cannot give you the name of a doctor or hospital that uses reflexology today. It is not allowed. Although many conscientious doctors are interested in this natural art of healing, they don't dare put it to use except on each other and their immediate families.

Dr. Clapp says, "I could give many case histories to show why I am so enthusiastic over zone therapy (reflexology). I never could have believed what it would do if I had not actually seen and done the work myself. I am more than delighted with it."

I know how Dr. Clapp felt, because in all the years I was practicing reflex massage, I never failed to be astonished at the miracles of healing it brought forth with nothing more than stimulating the reflexes with the fingers for a few minutes. It seemed like working magic, but, truly, I was only giving the magic of nature a helping hand in her efforts to release congested channels so that her healing forces could revive glandular activity.

22

A Journey Through the Alimentary Canal

Because the alimentary canal is the prime source of power which is converted and channeled where needed to keep the body functioning, it is important to understand how it operates. (See Diagram #1.)

With the help of the diagram, you can follow the long journey which food makes through the alimentary canal, or food canal, of your own body. The diagram is a reminder of the work which goes on in various parts of the canal, which will be helpful as you use reflexology to bring relief from any malfunction in this area.

YOUR SALIVARY GLANDS

First the food is cut up and ground by the action of the teeth, then pressed against the palate by the tongue. It is moistened and softened by the juices given off by the salivary glands. There are three different types of glands—those under the tongue, those near the jaw, and those near the inner ear—and each produces a different kind of salivary juice.

HOW GASTRIC JUICES ARE PRODUCED

Now, in a softened state, the food slides down the 10-inch gullet into the stomach. During its stay there, gastric juices, produced at the rate of over six pints a day, soften it still further until it reaches the consistency of a paste. From time to time, a valve opens and

DIAGRAM I

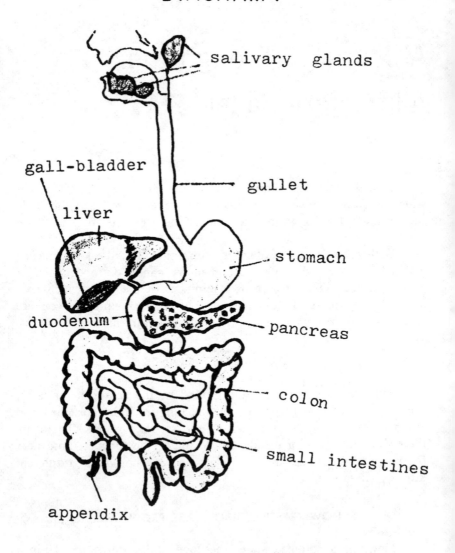

salivary glands

gall-bladder

gullet

liver

stomach

duodenum

pancreas

colon

small intestines

appendix

Diagram #1

134

allows small quantities of this paste to pass to the curving tube of the duodenum.

Two small pipes lead into the duodenum, one from the liver and another from the pancreas.

HOW THE LIVER FUNCTIONS

The liver, just below and to the right of the ribs, is the largest gland-organ in the whole body, weighing between three and four pounds, and it carries a complicated network of tiny bile canals and blood vessels. Each day, it produces about one and three-quarter pints of bile, most of which collects in the gall bladder before passing through the bile duct into the duodenum. One of the parts the liver plays in digestion is to help turn vegetable starch into animal starch, or glycogen.

HOW THE PANCREAS PRODUCES INSULIN

The pancreas, roughly oblong in shape, produces an alkaline fluid which helps to convert starch into sugar and solid fats into glycerides or fatty acids. It also produces insulin which controls the way the body makes use of sugar.

Soaked with bile and pancreatic juice, the food-paste now passes into the small intestine which itself produces close to a pint of digestive juices each day. The small intestine contains many small cone-like structures which act as pumps, extracting most of the usable part of the food-paste. It also has many muscles which expand and contract, pushing along the unusable food, much as the squeezing of a tube pushes along toothpaste.

Near the point where the food passes into the large intestine is an organ called the caecum, which ends in a kind of cul-de-sac called the appendix. The rising and descending parts of the large intestine are attached to the fleshy wall of the abdomen. The cross-wise part is suspended by means of a fold from the large membrane called peritoneum which envelops the whole of the intestines and the liver. The large intestine (colon) squeezes the unusable food along, extracting water from it on the way, toward the rectum and the anus where it is expelled from the body.

Since between 65 and 70 percent of an adult's weight is made up of water, the importance of consuming an adequate supply of water daily cannot be over-emphasized.

23

The Importance of the
Pancreas In Diabetes

If you are one of the many who are suffering from diabetes, you are aware that the malfunctioning of the pancreas is the cause of your disease.

The pancreas is one of the endocrine glands, roughly oblong in shape, and is the producer of insulin which controls the way the body makes use of sugar.

It consists mainly of a little group of gland cells linked to the duodenum by an extremely intricate system, as you can see in Diagram #1 in Chapter 22.

Most of its gland cells pour out juices which aid digestion. Set in the middle of the pancreatic tissue are small islands of different cells which produce a secretion called insulin, and this substance flows directly into the blood stream. It reaches all parts of the body and controls the body's use of sugar. If something goes wrong with the pancreas, these tiny islands quit working properly and the sugar in our blood increases and we become ill with the disease called diabetes mellitus. Scientists have shown that this disease frequently arises because of the lack of minute amounts of the hormone insulin from these vitally important gland cells. And hypoglycemia is caused by the opposite; when the pancreas is in malfunction it can also produce too much insulin, thus causing low blood sugar. Doctors are now learning that this is the root cause of many of our modern diseases.

**How to Stimulate the Pancreas with
Reflex Massage**

If you will look on Endocrine Gland Chart #3, in the front of this book, you can see how the pancreas lies almost in the center

of the body, but just a little to the right. It is about six inches long
and two to two-and-a-half inches wide, and lies behind the stomach.
If you look at Chart #2, you will see that the pancreas will be stimulated by any massage given to the reflexes in the center of the hand.
The position of the thumb in Figure 28-1 (Chapter 28) for kidney reflex massage will also work in massaging the pancreas: also the reflexes to the stomach as shown in Figure 21-1 (Chapter 21), with the
thumb on one hand pressing into the center of the opposite hand.
Be sure and massage the reflexes in both hands. Now, on Chart #1,
you can see how the meridian Zone Line 1 runs through the center
of the pancreas, so to use the reflex of the fingers to stimulate the
pancreas, you would massage the thumb and the two fingers next to
it, No. 1, No. 2, and No. 3. Remember that the location of the
reflexes in the hands are in the same position as the organs in the
body, while the meridian lines follow through the reflexes from the
fingers and toes.

If you use the Magic Reflex Massager, the pancreas reflexes
will get their share of massaging. If you are afflicted with diabetes,
then watch your insulin intake. Many times, this stimulates the
pancreas back into producing more of the natural insulin hormone
and your body will not require as much as you have been taking. If
you can awaken this endocrine gland back into normal function,
then you will no longer need the synthetic insulin. Only your doctor
can be the judge of this.

Remember, also, that the pancreas is related to the other six
endocrine glands, so do not neglect to stimulate the reflexes to all
of these hormone-producing glands. It is safe to use even on children,
although doctors claim there is no cure for many children afflicted
with this disease. Reflexology helps nature in her attempt to heal the
body by reactivating the vital life force back into these congested
areas.

I have seen some amazing things happen, which surprised me
many times, when the doctors said they couldn't be done. So, I say,
have faith in nature and massage your way back to health.

Dear Mrs. Carter:
    I have your book "Helping Yourself With Foot Reflexology"
and I think it is the best investment I have ever made in a book.
I think it is wonderful and I know it took a lot of your time to
compile this book. God love you for it. Thank you and God
bless you.
                                                    Mrs. V., Texas

24

Reflexology Helps
Hypoglycemia Victims

Millions of people are unaware that they are suffering from hypoglycemia (low blood sugar), which may masquerade as a neurosis and many other ailments.

In their book, "Low Blood Sugar and You", Carlton Fredericks, Ph.D., and Herman Goodman, M.D., give us some startling facts of how unaware millions are suffering from some form of hypoglycemia. They claim hypoglycemia is one of civilized man's most dangerous and most unrecognized illnesses, and tell us, "It has gone unidentified as a root cause of both minor and major physical and emotional problems for years."

An unbelievable array of symptoms is caused by low blood sugar. It can turn a balanced person into an apprehensive hypochondriac. It can make a psychiatric wreck out of a normal, well-adjusted individual. It creates intolerable anxiety. The symptoms of low blood sugar not only resemble neurosis or psychosis, they also perfectly imitate epilepsy, migraine headache, peptic ulcer, rheumatoid arthritis, insomnia, asthma, and other allergies. Low blood sugar can cause some of the "side reactions" blamed on drugs. It can directly cause alcoholism, and can possibly lead to drug addiction.

Dr. Herman Goodman and Carlton Fredericks tell us, "low blood sugar is too infrequently not detected in a complete medical checkup, and when it *is* recognized, the treatment prescribed for it by physicians, forty years behind the times, is the recommendation of more sugar, which is the opposite of what the patient needs, and makes every symptom worse."

We are all aware that glands may be normal, overactive, or underactive. This brings us up to the pancreas which we know to be one of the endocrine glands. If this gland is underactive, it causes diabetes. But few have ever given thought to what happens if the pancreas becomes *overactive*. A diabetic is given insulin to keep the blood sugar down to normal levels. We have all heard of the dramatic and disquieting results of taking too much insulin which causes the blood sugar to lower too much and too fast.

So what happens if the pancreas is overactive? It is producing too much insulin and is over-responsive to sugar. Many doctors mistakenly prescribe sugar for the hypoglycemic, which actually puts him in more danger than if he had diabetes. Many unsuspecting sufferers of low blood sugar walk around in insulin shock in a lesser or greater degree, not realizing what the trouble is.

This can be infinitely horrible—all the more so when the sufferer doesn't know what's wrong, and can't find out and winds up diagnosed as a neurotic, hypochondriac, eccentric, "nut," or a chronic invalid. Think of the thousands of poor souls whose lives have been ruined, when they may have only been suffering from a malfunctioning pancreas, and low blood sugar.

Seale Harris, M.D., says, "The low blood sugar of today is the diabetes of tomorrow."

HOW TO MASSAGE THE REFLEXES FOR HYPOGLYCEMIA

Now let us look to Reflexology to help us overcome this little understood, but dangerous, disease of our modern today. It doesn't matter if the gland is overactive or underactive. Reflex massage is the only medium which I know of that will enable the glands to return to their normal state of functioning, aside from proper diet as given in "Low Blood Sugar and You."

As I have explained in other chapters, the endocrine glands are all interrelated, so if the pancreas is in malfunction it is out of harmony with the other six hormone-producing endocrine glands. To help the sufferer of hypoglycemia, we will massage not only the reflexes to the pancreas, but the reflexes to the other endocrine glands as well.

By looking at Chart #3, you will see that the reflexes to the pancreas are located about in the center of both hands. So press and massage this area for a few minutes, and as you massage it you will also be giving the adrenal and the thymus glands their share of stimulation at the same time. All glands are important to correct the functioning of the pancreas. If you are using the Magic Reflex Massager, this will give an equal amount of stimulation as you roll it around in your hands.

Now let us go to the reflexes of the thyroid which are located just under the pad of the thumb, as shown in the illustration in the chapter on endocrine glands. This also may get some stimulation from the magic massager but usually needs a device which will reach in a little deeper, such as the hand massager, or you may use the knuckle of your finger to press in and massage. Keep pressing until you feel a tender spot, then massage it.

Now let us find the reflex to the pituitary which is located in the pad. of the thumb and is also shown in the chapter explaining the endocrine glands. Press into this area until you find a sore spot which may feel quite sharp when you touch it. You will probably have to use a device other than your fingers to reach into the reflex to this very important gland. After massaging it a few moments, we will turn to the reflexes to the gonads which hold their importance in keeping the whole body in balance.

On Chart #3, you will see how the reflexes to the testes and the ovaries (gonads) are located in the wrist on the side of the hand that the little finger (or 5th finger) is located. This is the area you will massage by using the thumb of the opposite hand as described in the chapter on endocrine glands. By pressing in to this area, you will find tender spots and this is where you will massage to bring the gonad glands into normal efficiency.

Reflexing the Liver for Hypoglycemia

Now that we have learned how to massage the reflexes to the endocrine glands in treating hypoglycemia, we will turn to the liver, an organ which also has an important share in the cause of hypoglycemia.

Remember that the reflex to the liver is located on the pad below the little finger on the right hand. Be sure and massage well in this whole area when there are symptoms of hypoglycemia. Also work on the webs, especially the one between the thumb and the first finger.

Hypoglycemia Masquerades
as Other Diseases

Many American medical men are painfully unaware that hypoglycemia is a common disorder that masquerades as half a hundred other diseases, according to Carlton Fredericks, Ph.D. and Herman Goodman, M.D.

How a Doctor Recovered after Three
Years of Illness

Doctor Stephen Gyland, tells of his experience of illness that lasted through three years of suffering, he says.

> If all physicians would read the work of Dr. Seale Harris, . . . thousands of persons would not have to go through what I did. I was examined by 14 specialists and three nationally known clinics before a diagnosis was made by a six-hour glucose (sugar) tolerance test. Previous diagnoses having been brain tumor, diabetes, and cerebral arteriosclerosis. . . . Since then I have used this hard-earned knowledge in diagnosis and curing the condition in numerous patients.

If you or any one you know seems to have an illness which has not been correctly diagnosed, think of hypoglycemia. Don't depend completely on reflexology, demand a six-hour glucose test. Then, with the proper sugar-free diet, let reflexology revitalize the malfunctioning glands back to normal, thus bringing harmony and health back into your *whole* body.

MUSCULAR DYSTROPHY

How A Victim of Muscular Dystrophy Was Helped in Minutes

When we were on a trip up the Northwest Channel of Canada, on a ferry, I noticed a quite attractive lady dragging her foot as she walked, her husband having to help her most of the time even though I could tell it hurt her to be so dependent on him. Some time later my husband joined her husband in a game of cards, so I went over and sat beside her. It wasn't long until she was telling me of her troubles.

Mrs. M. said that she had muscular dystrophy and the doctors told her there wasn't anything that could be done for her, and she would just have to be reconciled to becoming an invalid as the disease would progress slowly over her whole body. She was understandably depressed and very unhappy.

I asked her if she had ever heard of reflexology and she said that she hadn't. I told her a little about how it worked and asked her to let me massage her hand, which I did for about ten minutes and she was amazed at the results. She couldn't wait to tell her husband about it and how good it made her feel all over. I offered to give her a complete treatment later if she wanted me to do so. We made an appointment to meet them in their stateroom where I massaged her hands and feet for about 20 minutes. We made a date to have dinner with them later.

When they came into the dining room, she was walking alone without a sign of a limp, and her face was radiant. When the girl who was sharing their stateroom with them came in, she looked at Mrs. M. and asked what had happened to her. She was amazed at what they told her about Reflexology.

Mrs. M. said that she was starved for the first time in months. Mr. M. and she could not believe the results that they were seeing happening before their very eyes in such a short period of time. And once again I thanked God for leading me to this wonderful method of bringing health to my fellow man.

This natural method of healing is safe and free for all to use. I hope you will put it to work to help not only yourself, but also to help others who are sent to you for relief from suffering and need the freedom from illness and pain.

How Reflexology Helped Multiple Sclerosis Victim

"I started using reflexology treatments on my husband and myself, then it really grew out of hand. All of my acquaintances wanted me to massage their feet.

"God led me to a 39-year-old woman suffering from multiple sclerosis. This method hasn't performed a miracle because only God can, but she is comfortable. Before treatments, she had to have shots in her knees. Her menstrual periods had stopped. Her skin was very scaly. Her bowels weren't performing. Happy to say, all these are cleared up. I have only been treating her a year, twice a week. She had been bed-ridden for 13 years before I met her.

"I am sorry, but I have become disillusioned with the Medical Profession as a whole—very few old, good M.D.'s left."

Mrs. D.A.

25

Alcoholism and Drug Addiction Considered Glandular Disorders

"Can you help alcoholism?" is the cry of so many as they reach hopeless hands out of the darkness of despair.

Yes, reflexology can help those who are lost in the clutches of alcohol or drugs. These words should be like the tolling of a bell ringing out a new hope of freedom to thousands of sufferers from either devastating disease, especially alcoholism. There are few diseases that can bring as much distress into the lives of the victims and their families as can alcoholism.

HOW MALFUNCTIONING ADRENAL GLANDS
ARE TO BLAME

In his book, *The Encyclopedia of Common Diseases,* J. I. Rodale says:

"Alcoholism is a glandular disorder, and we can compare it with diabetes, as neither can properly metabolize carbohydrates. In the case of diabetics, not enough insulin is produced by the pancreatic gland which has this function, so the patient suffers from high blood sugar.

In the case of alcoholics, *there is too much insulin* rather than too little, with the result that the alcoholic has low blood sugar. What causes the extra insulin that causes the low blood sugar? Apparently, the function of at least two glands is involved—the *adrenals* (it is the cortex or covering of these glands that is involved), and the *pituitary* which regulates the adrenals.

E. M. Abrahamson, M.D., in his book, *Body, Mind and Sugar,* says.

> Alcoholism is caused by a deficiency in the adrenal cortical hormones — those hormones whose action is antithetical to insulin.
>
> The trouble may not be in the adrenal cortical itself, however, but in the master gland, the pituitary, which for some reason fails to stimulate the adrenal cortical glands as it does in normal operation of the endocrine system. It is believed, moreover, that this disability of the pituitary is *not* caused by the alcoholism itself but antedates its development.
>
> Hyperinsulinism, with its chronic partial blood sugar starvation, is an essential underlying cause of alcoholism.

If what these experts say is true, then we know that by energizing the vital life force into the endocrine system with *Reflexology,* we can help nature return these glands back into normal functioning, thus helping the person who is afflicted with alcoholism return to a normal life.

HOW TO HELP THE ALCOHOLIC WITH REFLEXOLOGY

After reading the above explanation of the cause of alcoholism, we can see that we must first concentrate on the reflexes to the pituitary gland which are located in the center of the pad on both thumbs.

After massaging these, move down to the adrenal reflexes in the center of the hands, as shown in Figure 28-1 in Chapter 28, and massage these a few minutes. Also massage the reflexes to the pancreas and liver. (See Chart #2.)

You will probably find the reflexes to these glands quite tender at first, so be gentle in the beginning.

After working on the reflexes to the pituitary and adrenal glands, the pancreas and liver, for about five minutes, you can move on to the reflexes to the rest of the endocrine glands. Study the chart on endocrine glands (#3).

Be sure to give each of these reflexes your special attention, since we have learned that if one of these important hormone-producing glands is out of balance, it will throw all of the others out of harmony. Remember, when this system is in perfect order, so will the whole body be able to adjust back to a normal functioning of all glands and organs.

Alcoholism Is a Much Misunderstood Disease

Alcoholism is a disease which is not understood as such. Wives and husbands nag, children weep, doctors scold, and the bars get richer, and through it all the agonized and helpless alcoholic suffers more shame, pain, and bewilderment than anyone involved.

Reflexology Gives New Hope to the Alcoholic

So let us not condemn, but hold out a helping hand and show them that the answer lies *in their own hands.*

Just by massaging the reflexes to certain glands, every person who is afflicted with the disease of alcoholism may return to a normal state, free of his craving for alcoholic stimulants.

TREATING DRUG WITHDRAWAL WITH REFLEXOLOGY

Just as there is new hope for the alcoholic, reflexology offers a way back for the drug addict.

It has been discovered that by inserting an electric needle in the lobe of the ear of a drug addict he returns to normal without the pain of withdrawal symptoms.

Reflexology can be used to accomplish the same results, by holding a tight pressure on certain reflex points in the lobes of the ears for a period of five to ten minutes or more; then relax the pressure. Repeat this for as long as needed, or until the patient recovers and feels he has no more need of the treatment.

Devices May Be Used to Exert Pressure

Various devices may be used to exert pressure on the ear lobes. Clothespins might be too tight for this tender area, but the reflex clamps could be used; or pressure with the fingers if one has the patience to hold this position for the length of time needed. The patient can easily use this latter method on himself by pressing each ear lobe with the tips of his thumb and forefinger, even digging the fingernails in if he feels it necessary.

Other Benefits of Reflexology

The techniques of reflexology can be helpful to the person trying to recover from an occasional hangover, such as the social drinker who has over-indulged and would like a quick and painless recovery.

It can also be helpful to those who are trying to withdraw from the habit of heavy drinking before they succumb to the life of an alcoholic.

As reflexology restores the glands and organs to normalcy, your body will once more become a melody of beauty and balance free of all abnormal cravings.

26

Reflexing the Appendix and Ileocecal Valve

While it is true fewer people are dying from appendicitis, the number of people who suffer from this disease is the same as ever. The *Pfizer Spectrum,* a drug trade magazine, reports that appendectomies are still the most frequently performed operations in the general hospital.

Acute appendicitis attacks are sudden, give little forewarning, and the diagnosis is complicated even for your doctor.

HELPING APPENDICITIS WITH REFLEXOLOGY

In using reflex massage to the appendix, let us look at Figure 26. See how the thumb is pressed into the side of the right hand about half way toward the wrist under the little finger. If this spot is tender when you press on it firmly, then it could be an indication of a congested appendix. Massage this spot by digging the edge of the thumb in with a press and roll motion. If the symptoms do not subside in a few minutes after massaging, ice packs should be applied and your doctor contacted, if an attack is indicated. Otherwise, you may massage these reflexes as long as you wish.

You will see on Zone Chart #1 that the meridian lines 3 and 4 would run through the appendix, so to help nature further in her effort to revive glandular activity, work on the middle and ring fingers, third and fourth reflex. Reflex clamps or rubber bands may be used on these fingers and pressing with the reflex comb can also be of help in holding a steady pressure on the reflex to the appendix.

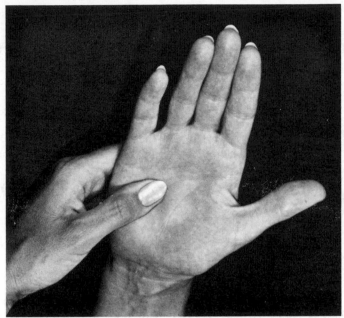

Figure 26-1. Position for massaging the reflexes to the appendix and the ileocecal valve.

If the tenderness does not lessen in two or three days, there may be an indication of pus and you should have the attention of your chiropractor or doctor to make sure there is no immediate danger.

ALLERGIES AND THE ILEOCECAL VALVE

Because the reflexes to this little valve are located in almost the same place as the appendix, it will be treated with the same massage technique in the same place. Usually, tenderness in this area of the right hand, and also on the foot, will indicate that there is inflammation of the ileocecal valve instead of the appendix. It will probably take longer to massage this area and dissipate the inflammation.

How to Overcome Allergies

This is the button you will press if you are trying to overcome allergies of any kind. It was found that this valve was red and inflamed in every case of allergy when operations were performed on accident victims.

These reflexes can take a lot of massaging without any harm; so *if it is sore, rub it out!*

Reflexology Used 33 Years

Dear Mildred Carter:

Reflexology is not new to me, for I have been using it 33 years, not professionally, but on myself. It will do all you say it can do.

I'm never sick and never see a doctor, use no drugs of any kind.

Thank you,
L.M.W.

Reflex Cures Condition of 40 Years

Gentlemen:

On March 4th of this year you sent me a copy of Mrs. Carter's book—Helping Yourself with Foot Reflexology.

I think you should know that it is the best investment I ever made in my life. I will not bore you with the gruesome details, but it effected a cure of a condition with which I have been troubled for over 40 years.

Thankfully,
Mrs. H.M.B., Ohio

Dear Mrs. Carter:

I let my daughter take my book on Reflexology. I want another one. I had such good results by using your book on myself. I was nearly crippled with something in my hip and leg, down to my knee and had spent nearly $150 on doctors, and didn't get much relief until I got your book on Reflexology. But now I am all right.

Thanks to you,
Mrs. A.S.M.

27

How Reflexology Can
Heal Hemorrhoids

I explained in my earlier book, "Helping Yourself With Foot Reflexology," how you would find the reflexes to the rectum located along the bony edge of the heel. If you have hemorrhoids, you will find a sore spot in this area. When the soreness is massaged out, the hemorrhoids will also vanish.

Since hemorrhoids are swollen veins in the rectum, we will look at Chart #2 and Chart #1 and see how the meridian line 1 goes through the rectum. We will, therefore, work mainly on the reflexes in the thumbs. You will also work the thumb of one hand around the bony edge of the opposite hand just above the wrist. Use the press and roll method as you try to feel out the tender spots; then change to the other hand and massage it in the same way. You will probably find that the tenderness will be on just one side due to the fact that the swollen vein is usually on the side, rather than in the center of the rectum.

Now, take the thumb and massage up the center of the wrist about one-third of the distance to the elbow, using this same method of massage on both hands.

VICTIMS OF HEMORRHOIDS SUFFER IN SILENCE

Hemorrhoids are one of the most painful conditions and are usually suffered in silence by those who have them, yet they are among the quickest to respond to treatments by reflexology.

Hemorrhoids, (commonly known as piles) are nothing more than congested veins. They are the cause of much suffering and inconvenience. At times, they may protrude and cause excessive bleeding.

Pain of Hemorrhoids Stopped in Minutes

I can tell you of many cases in which the pain of hemorrhoids was stopped in minutes, and the amazing fact is that all indications of the offending irritation vanished completely, never to return—this in some of the most severe cases.

Although men do suffer with hemorrhoids, there are far more women afflicted with this painful and embarrassing complaint.

The method that has given the quickest and most successful results in treating hemorrhoids is through the reflexes on the feet.

How to Use Tongue Probe to Relieve Hemorrhoids

We will now turn to the technique of the tongue probe which you learned in a previous chapter. Since the rectum is in the first zone, you can see by looking at Charts #1 and #2 how the reflexes in the tongue will affect the hemorrhoids. The method of tongue pressure is the same in all cases. Using the handle of a tablespoon or a tongue probe, press down on the center of the tongue as far back as possible and hold it from two to ten minutes.

I can tell you of hundreds of cases who have been relieved from the pain of hemorrhoids in minutes by pressing the reflex buttons on the sides of the heels of the feet alone, and many more who have used the massage of the reflex in the hands and the tongue pressure technique. You may have to move the probe into different positions to find the right spot as there may be more than one congested vein, as explained in the chapter on the tongue. It may also take some practice to use the tongue pressure technique without gagging. You can also get results by clamping the fingers or using pressure with the comb or the fingers to activate these hemorrhoid reflexes into sending nature's healing life force into the congested vein in the rectum.

I am writing this chapter on hemorrhoids for all who have suffered in silence for these many years. You will learn the best method for your particular case and be able to use it immediately when pain strikes.

Reflexology Helps Prolapsed Rectum

A prolapsed rectum is another condition which can cause untold agony. As a person gets older, this condition can get worse. The rectum is often badly swollen and very much inflamed and protrudes more and more. The benefit of reflex massage is almost unbelievable for this serious condition. You will use the same method that you used for the hemorrhoid disorder, since this involves the same area.

When you use the above techniques of reflex massage, you are sending the healing forces of nature to revive activity into the whole lower lumbar area.

I suffered from hemorrhoids for years and at times there was such excessive bleeding, I thought I would bleed to death. Many times, I would get up and work all night because the pain was so severe I couldn't lie down or sit still. I used every kind of an ointment there was. The doctor didn't see anything very seriously wrong. Since I wouldn't take drugs, I suffered in silence; piles are something you don't talk about.

How Reflexology Helped the Author

I was introduced to reflexology by a friend of my cousin who was visiting at her home. She was kind enough to give me a treatment. When she touched the reflexes to the hemorrhoids on my heels, I nearly went through the ceiling from the pain. She showed me how to find these buttons so I could massage them myself. "You will never be bothered with hemorrhoids again if you massage all of the tenderness out of the reflexes in this area," she promised. I thanked her, but can truthfully say that I doubted her word even though I was amazed at the great feeling of stimulation I felt after the treatment. I did massage the soreness out as she had instructed, "in just two or three days," and I have never had a recurrence of the disorder in these many years since. I also have never stopped using reflexology.

This encounter with reflexology led to my study of the amazing methods of this natural art of healing and my study and research continue to this day.

28

Helping the Kidneys and
Bladder with Reflex Massage

You will find the adrenal glands located next to the pancreas. There are two adrenal glands, one attached to the top of each kidney. By looking at Charts #2 and #3, in the front of this book, you will see how they lie on each side of the body just under the spleen. You will also notice that the reflexes to the kidneys are almost in the center of the hand. If you look at a picture of the body drawn to scale of the internal organs, you will see how they are crowded one behind the other.

Your kidneys are two little filtering systems lying on each side of the spine. Sometimes you hear of people donating one of their kidneys to another person because both of his kidneys were deteriorating. No one can live without at least one kidney to filter poison out of the body. I wonder how many such operations might be avoided if reflex massage were used to help nature reactivate circulation of the vital life force back into these malfunctioning organs. It would do no harm to give reflexology a chance before more drastic measures are taken.

Look at the charts in the front of this book and notice how the reflex to the kidneys lies just about in the center of the hand, while in the body chart you can see that they are located on each side of the spine. Be sure to massage the reflexes to the kidneys on both hands. Notice how the thumb is placed in the center of the hand in Figure 28-1. Massage this area by using the pressing and rolling method. If the kidneys are badly affected, then only massage this for a very few seconds the first time. If you look at the Zone Chart #1, you will see

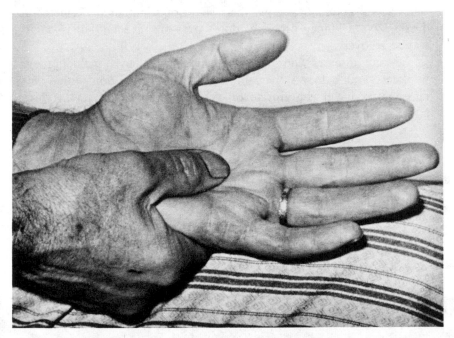

Figure 28-1. Position for massaging the reflexes to the adrenal gland and kidneys.

how the lines from #2 and #3 fingers run through the kidneys. You can also help in their fight for life by massaging the reflexes on these two fingers. Search for tender spots on both the front and the sides, pressing from the tips to the base. When you find a tender spot in this area, assume that it is a kidney reflex and work it out. Since we are going to need all the stimulation we can get to reactivate the healing forces back into these organs, you might also work on the same reflexes in the feet. Be sure not to *over-massage* these reflexes to the kidneys until they are on their way back to functioning normally.

HOW REFLEXOLOGY CAN HELP YOUR KIDNEYS

Nature's tendency is to restore all normal conditions in the body when we give her the necessary help by stimulating the circulation of the vital life force with reflex massage. When the Magic Reflex Massager or the Rollo Reflex Massager is used in this area, the kidney reflexes will automatically get their share of stimulation. Remember, if you have a kidney problem, don't over-massage until it is on its way to recovery.

Many diseases can be laid to faulty kidneys, including eye weakness and kidney stones. In treating this condition with reflex massage, you will concentrate on relaxing the urinary tract, which is the excretory duct leading from the kidneys to the bladder. By referring to Chart #2, you can see where the location of the bladder is in conjunction to the kidneys. In Figure 28-1, you can see how to massage the kidney and Figure 28-2 shows the position for massaging the bladder.

You will massage between these two areas, back and forth on the ureter reflex, relaxing the tension so nature can eliminate the kidney stones and other congestion through normal muscular contraction.

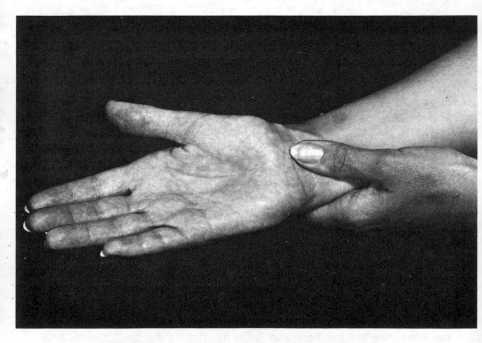

Figure 28-2. Shows position for massaging the reflexes to the lower lumbar area and the bladder.

Always be sure to massage the reflexes in both hands, especially for the kidneys. Never unbalance nature by leaving one side untuned.

How Kidneys Are Helped with Reflex Devices

The tongue probe (explained in another chapter) also works very well in stimulating the bladder reflexes. *Be sure you are not pregnant,* as pressing on the back of the tongue could cause a *miscarriage,* as described in the chapter on childbirth.

Using the reflex comb with the teeth pressed across the kidney reflexes will also be of great benefit. Clamping the ends of fingers 1, 2 and 3 will also give nature added help in healing any congestion or malfunction in this area. Keep in mind that pressure relaxes, and massage stimulates and heals. Nature needs both in her efforts to bring the balance of harmony back into your system.

Man Passes Stone in Ten Minutes

Dear Mrs. Carter,

I have to write and tell you what happened to me after I received your book. I started to use the directions about massaging the reflexes in my feet, and in about ten minutes I went to the bathroom and passed a stone. It was big enough to make a noise when it hit the water. I didn't even know I had any stones. I guess you know what I think of your wonderful book. I feel great thanks to you.

W.M., Kansas City, Mo.

REFLEX MASSAGE FOR BLADDER TROUBLES

You have already located the bladder and its reflexes on the charts in the front of this book, but let us refer back to Charts #1 and #2 once more. Notice how the reflexes to the bladder are located in the lower part of the hand and the position of the thumb on this area in Figure 28-2. If the bladder is congested or affected in any way, you will find these reflexes quite tender. Massage this with the usual press and roll of the thumb, working the area shown in Chart #2 and also down onto the wrist area of the lower lumbar reflexes.

By relaxing tension and breaking up congestion with reflex

massage, I have had many wonderful results in helping cases of bladder troubles. When you stimulate these reflexes, you are allowing normal circulation to flow through the cells as nature intended. Look also to other glands which many times are the real cause of bladder trouble. If you find tender reflexes in any area which is sending out a cry for help, *massage it out.*

Since the bladder is in the center of your body, clamps on fingers 1, 2, and 3 can also be very beneficial in helping nature relax and heal any congestion in the bladder area.

However, do not neglect to see your chiropractor, naturopath, or doctor as the infection might be of a more serious nature that needs his attention. Remember, today's chiropractor has to put in more actual hours of schooling than do medical doctors; yet, he practices only natural methods of healing, using no shots, harmful drugs, or operations. Nevertheless, he keeps a personal interest in your health and well being. Many chiropractors now use reflexology in their practice to give their patients every advantage of receiving all the benefits of natural healing.

Reflexologist from India Gives History of Healings

Mr. Th., a very successful reflexologist in Arizona, studied reflexology in India and has a unique and successful way of massaging the reflexes to help nature promote healing of malfunctioning parts of the body. He was aided back to walking after being told that he would never walk again. He was also helped to better vision by the use of reflexology.

I will let Mr. Th. tell you in his own words how he helped one lady.

The other night I was treating a lady who has had several treatments, only on this particular night she had obtained a nasty cut from a rose thorn. I worked all around it on the right foot then I went to the pituituary reflex on the left foot. After a second or two I asked her to wet her finger with saliva from her own mouth and put it on the cut on her right foot. Then I continued the treatment. After the treatment I asked her to look at the sore. To her amazement there was nothing there but a red mark, like those left when you peel a scab from an old cut.

Mr. TH.—J.

Mrs. Th. adds—Reflexology has helped me with a bladder problem (since childhood) which was very embarrassing, to say the least. Also Reflexology has rid me of the pain in my bunion which I had thought would be with me to the grave. It pained 24 hours a day.

Mrs. TH.—J.

29

How to Treat Arthritis with Reflexology

Arthritis is only a new name for rheumatism which has caused suffering throughout the ages. We now know that it attacks in many forms. The most common types are rheumatoid arthritis and osteo-arthritis. Together they are responsible for over 90 percent of all cases of arthritis.

It is now known as a degenerative disease, and official medicine admits its inability to penetrate the mysteries of arthritis and find a cure for it even though it is the most agonizing and crippling disease of the 20th century. There are over thirteen million arthritis sufferers in the United States. It is one of the fastest growing of all degenerative diseases.

The body is a wonderful work of art which no man can duplicate. It takes years and years of abuse and neglect to bring about the eventual breakdown of this intricate system. Then people wonder why they start having aches and pains when they should be at the very peak of health. "Just when I could start enjoying life," they say, "this had to happen to me."

Fortunately, however, we can treat arthritis at any stage with simple reflex massage, restoring lost functioning and alleviating pains and aches, and halting further damage to one's system.

HOW ARTHRITIS AFFECTS THE WHOLE BODY

The most serious form of arthritis is called *rheumatoid arthritis.* It is extremely painful and a crippling disease which affects people of

160

all ages, particularly young adults. Women are afflicted with rheumatoid arthritis three times as often as men.

Paavo O. Airola, N.C., writes in his book, *There Is A Cure for Arthritis:*

> It is important to realize that although swollen and inflamed joints may seem to be the very first signals of approaching arthritis, they are not at all the first symptoms of the onset of the disease. Arthritis is not a local disease of a particular joint but a systemic disorder, a disease which affects the entire body. The arthritis patient usually suffers from a general deterioration of health in the form of sluggishness in the function of his vital organs; incomplete digestion and assimilation of food; nutritional deficiencies; glandular disorders, *particularly in the endocrine system;* impaired elimination of metabolic wastes and toxins; and a weakened nervous system and circulation. These systemic disturbances affect the biochemical structure of the various tissues of the body and cause what one of the pioneer practitioners of biological medicine in the United States, R. P. Watterson, M.D., calls a "biochemical suffocation."

HOW YOU CAN RELIEVE ARTHRITIS

When using reflex massage, we are opening the channels in all parts of the body and we can readily see why people are having such wonderful results when they use reflex massage to help arthritis. Every time a reflex button is pressed, it instantly sends a charge of magnetic vital life force surging through the body to the particular area with which it is in contact, opening and stimulating the channel as it goes. When you press many reflex buttons, you can picture what is happening all through your body's network of intricate channels. No wonder you feel so exhilarated with renewed life and vitality immediately after a reflex treatment! You have released the clogged channels, leaving no place of biochemical suffocation.

The Importance of the Endocrine System

The first *glands* you should concentrate on are the endocrine glands, and then follow through on the rest of the glands until you have covered the reflexes to the whole body.

Once we realize that our glandular system is the transmitter of life forces which are transformed into function through the body, we can readily understand the importance of using reflex massage to stimulate the transmission pattern of the body's electrical network.

So, let us take a quick look at Endocrine Charts #3 and #1. Notice how the lines run from fingers #1 and #2 on down through all of the endocrine glands especially, ending in toes #1 and #2. You can see why you should concentrate on the thumb and first finger, and also the third finger to some extent.

The Importance of Your Pituitary Gland

Since the pituitary is the king gland, you should start massaging the center of the pad on the thumb as shown in Figure 5-1; then move on to the pineal reflex, which is located just a little toward the inside of the thumb.

If you find a tender spot in either of these places, you will be sure you are on the right track.

You may massage these reflex buttons either with the rolling-pressing motion or by holding a solid pressure on them. You can do this with the tip of the finger, or the fingernail of the same hand, thus pressing both reflexes at the same time; or, massage with the fingers of the opposite hand; or, use the massage clamps as shown in Figure 10-2, as they can be used on more than one finger at a time and held for a longer period of time.

You can see on Chart #2 how important it is to work on all of the fingers on both hands.

Following down Endocrine Chart #3, we next come to the thyroid and parathyroids.

Massaging the Thyroid and Parathyroid Glands

To stimulate these important glands, we press in to the reflexes under the ball of the thumb as shown in Figure 15-1 and Figure 5 in the front of the book, using the thumb of the opposite hand or the Hand Massager shown in Figure 5-1. The Magic Massager will stimulate the thyroids since it reaches into all the glands which have reflexes in the palm of the hand. As the thyroid is in the center of the body, you will work on the reflexes in both hands.

Massaging the Thymus

Now we move down to the thymus on Chart #3. The full importance of this little gland is not yet known but since it is one of the endocrine glands we know that it has its place in affecting arthritis.

As you can see on Chart #2, its reflexes are so centrally located that it gets its share of massage whenever the palm of the hand is massaged.

Massaging the Pancreas and Adrenal Glands

Let us look at the pancreas on Chart #3, and see how it lies over the adrenal glands. Since the reflexes to these endocrine glands are in the same area, you should press into the center of the palm of the hand to massage the reflexes to them. Press the thumb into the center of the hand, using a rolling and pressing motion. Since these reflexes in the center of the palm are more sensitive than most of the other reflexes, you won't need a hard pressure here. The Magic Massager will cover these reflexes quite satisfactorily if you have one.

And keep in mind that the reflexes in the palm are going to activate the more sensitive organs and glands in your body, *so you must not over massage for the first two weeks*. Just massage for two or three minutes on each hand every other day for the first week.

REACTIVATING YOUR REPRODUCTIVE SYSTEM

Now we move to the gonads—ovaries in women, the testes in men. These are the organs of reproduction, but they also produce hormones that create the inner warmth in our system, preventing all tendencies for inflexibility, hardening, and stiffening. No wonder they play such an important part in arresting the development of arthritis!

You will notice on your Chart #3 that the reflexes to these all-important glands are located on the lower part of the hand and on down into the wrist area.

To give these glands the proper amount of massage, use the thumb of the opposite hand and massage the whole area of the wrist starting under the little finger and working over to the center of the wrist. If you hold your hand up with the back toward you, this would be the outside of the hand, the same as the outside of the foot on which these glands are located under the ankle.

How to Stimulate the Liver

Now let us look once more at the reflex to the liver, which is located in the right hand. You will notice in Chart #2 how the reflexes to the liver and other organs are crowded into a small area in the hand, so when you are massaging the reflex to one gland, you will unavoidably also massage the reflexes to several glands in the near area.

Place the thumb of the left hand on the pad under the little finger on the right hand, and use the pressing and rolling motion of massaging; and don't forget to massage the web between the thumb and first finger, working on any tender button you may find here.

Lungs Need Reflex Massage

Now let us go to the area under the fingers and massage this whole area clear down into the pads located in the upper third of the palm, where the lung reflexes are located. Don't forget to massage this reflex on both hands.

Reflex Massage for Stomach

To find the stomach reflexes, the thumb is pressed into the soft spot from the web on toward the center of the hand as explained in Chapter 21 on the stomach. Be sure to massage both hands.

Massage All Reflexes in Hands

Work through the reflexes of the whole hand in this way. Massage *all the reflexes* in both hands, not forgetting to search for tender buttons in the webs between all the fingers, keeping in mind that by activating just one tiny pinpoint in your reflexes you can send an electrical charge of vital force into a clogged channel, releasing a king-pin that has been the cause of all your trouble.

Since arthritis is caused by metabolic disorder and systemic disturbances, particularly in glandular activity, which bring about pathological biochemical changes in all the tissues of the body, we can easily understand why so many victims of this dreaded disease are getting such astonishing results when they reactivate the whole glandular system with reflex massage.

How a Ranch Woman Recovered from
Arthritis

A very kind friend of the author's tries to help everyone she meets, no matter what their problems. She tells of a close neighbor on an adjoining ranch. She watched this woman become ill with arthritis, spreading over her body little by little, becoming helpless, no longer able even to enjoy walking outside on her ranch.

Visitor from France Brings Reflexology

Then she tells of the unexpected way in which she was introduced to my book on Foot Reflexology, which was brought by the relative of another neighbor who was visiting from France. She immediately sent for one and started to study it. She asked the friend afflicted with arthritis if she wanted her to try the massage on her, since it could do no harm.

Mrs. M. says that her neighbor seemed to feel improvement the first day they tried reflex massage. The first night she said she slept the whole night through without waking once.

Anyone familiar with reflex massage knows this is usually the first sign that they are receiving benefit from the treatments—the feeling of relaxation and being able to sleep soundly through the night. Remember the body heals while we sleep—this is why doctors give drugs to help you sleep. Reflex massage, instead of making you feel drugged when you wake up, gives you the feeling of renewed vitality and pep.

Mrs. M. tells us of the surprisingly quick recovery of her neighbor:

> Today she can walk as well as I can, resuming her help with the outside work on the ranch with joy, thanks to Reflexology.

30

How You Can Abort a Cold and Stop Coughs

The knowledge of the healing principles of reflexology is spreading throughout the world, following in the footsteps of the much exploited acupuncture, and the time is not too far distant when everyone will be able to cure coughs and colds for himself, without the dangers of medications.

If you have a bad cough, then try the finger massage first by pressing on the thumb and first and second fingers. These reflexes may be stimulated by a steady pressure held on them for about ten minutes at a time, unless you are using the rubber bands, in which case you will have to remove them as soon as the fingers start to turn blue. The reflex clamp can be used here with good advantage. Remember that the throat is located in the first zone which is the thumb; this is why we concentrate on the thumb and the fingers next to it for any problems of the throat. Next we would use the tongue probe to press on the reflexes on the center of the tongue with the handle of a knife or spoon or tongue probe for five or ten minutes.

I have cured many sore throats by just massaging under the big toe, and around the thumb.

How a Friend Was Cured of a Cold

I went to visit a dear friend and found her in bed suffering from a bad cold and a very sore throat. Her fever was high but she had refused to let anyone call a doctor.

I immediately went to work, first applying spring clothespins to the ends of all her fingers since I had nothing better with me.

I next fixed old-fashioned onion poultices and put them on her chest and her back. Then I uncovered her feet and went to work massaging all of the area around the big toe and the toes next to it. I especially concentrated on massaging the reflexes to the pituitary gland located in the center of the big toe and also in the center of the pad of the thumb. The rest of the reflexes I left alone as her body was trying to throw off enough poisons without stirring up more for it to take care of.

In less than an hour, J. was feeling much better and fell into a natural sleep, not waking until the next morning. Her fever had dropped to almost normal before I left for home. The next day, much against my advice, J. was up doing her work, feeling fine, except for being a little weak. She still says I was sent to save her life that day I made an unexpected visit.

How Doctor Fitzgerald Cured Whooping Cough in Five Minutes

The benefits of this reflex therapy are so powerful that it has cured many cases of the dreaded whooping cough in the days before vaccinations. Whooping cough is still not unheard of and it behooves everyone to learn the simple remedy by the use of reflex massage.

Dr. Wm. Fitzgerald, tells us:

Whooping cough is one of the simplest and most easily-cured diseases with which zone therapy (reflexology) has to contend. An ordinary case of whooping cough, which has persisted for weeks, can sometimes be cured in from three to five minutes. Rarely are more than four or five treatments necessary. After the application of a probe held down firmly on the back of the throat, little patients who had whooped themselves into a state of nervous and physical exhaustion never had another paroxysm of coughing.

Dr. Fitzgerald offered to demonstrate the method on one or one hundred cases and prove that in one to a half dozen treatments, whooping cough can be effectively and permanently overcome.

The doctor stated, "In the several cases of whooping cough treated, we have not yet seen a failure from the proper application of zone therapy (reflexology)."

How a Woman Stopped a Stranger's Cough

Mrs. L. tells of going into town to do her shopping and noticed a woman standing by her car coughing. "She seemed to be coughing rather hard. I was concerned but didn't like to be bold so I went on into the store. When I came out about 15 minutes later, the woman was still standing in the same place coughing harder than ever. After putting my groceries in the car I went over to her and said, 'Would you like to have me tell you how to stop that cough?' She looked at me hopelessly and shook her head 'yes' as she continued the paroxysm of coughing.

"I told her to place her thumb on the lower joint of the first finger and to press hard. She looked at me kind of queerly but followed my directions. The cough seemed to subside almost immediately. I waited a few minutes to make sure it didn't start again, then I left. The last I saw of the woman she was still standing in the same spot holding her finger."

Trachea (Wind Pipe) and How it Works

Let us look at the rest of your respiratory system which consists of two large tubes, one for each lung, leading off the trachea (or wind pipe) which taper on down into smaller bronchi tubes to make a tree-like formation within the lungs. You can see how disastrous it is for the body when a severe infection of these muscular bronchi results in destruction of the muscle necessary for contraction.

You will stimulate this part of your respiratory system as you massage the reflexes for the lungs and the voice. For special treatment of this area, you should concentrate on the thumb and first finger and tongue pressure.

Don't Over-Massage for Colds

A cold is nature's way of cleaning house; I mean eliminating the system of acid. It is trying to rid the body of accumulated poisons, through mucous membranes in the head, the nose, the sinuses and through the pores of the skin. If your system is in perfect order, you will not be susceptible to colds or the various types of flu and viruses which spread through the country every few months. Do you ever wonder why some people catch everything that comes along and others seem to be happily immune, and are never sick?

If you are one of these who never catch anything, then your body is not so burdened with poisons. But if you do have colds frequently, then your body is overburdened trying to eliminate toxic poisons, so you will not add further to its efforts to throw off accumulated poison by massaging all of the reflexes at this time. By concentrating on massaging the reflexes in the fingers and in the lung area, you will be giving nature a little help instead of hindrance in clearing up your cold. You may give kidneys a very short massage to help them in their work of eliminating these poisons the cold is trying to throw off, and the pituitary gland in the thumbs may be worked on in case of fever.

How Reflexology Saved Child from Rheumatic Fever

Mr. A. reports how he saved his daughter from the after-affects of rheumatic fever. "When Sally first became ill I didn't think too much about it," says Mr. A. "She had had a sore throat for a few days; her mother was away taking care of her sister in another state. Sally, the boys, and I always got along fine for a few days without her. But when Sally started to run a high fever I became panic-stricken. I called the family doctor who is one of those rare physicians who still makes house calls. When he arrived, he took one look at Sally and said, 'Strep throat, which could cause rheumatic fever and damage her heart, if her fever ran too high.' He gave me some medication and warned me to watch her closely, and if the fever went higher to call him immediately. And he said I had better call her mother. I put in an emergency call to Mrs. A. and when I told her of our troubles she wasn't one bit upset. Mary was always a sensible girl and knew how to keep her cool, as the boys say. 'Sally is all right,' She told me calmly, 'You use reflexology on her and the fever will go down.' Reflexology had become a by-word in our house where sickness was concerned. Mary's mother had used it to keep her family healthy for many years, having learned it from a neighbor. I felt the tensions of fear lift and I asked her what she wanted me to do. 'Massage the reflexes to the pituitary to take the fever down,' she said. 'This is the little spot that is so sore in the center of your big toe a lot of times.' I knew the spot! 'Also work on the thumb and web of both hands. But keep at it, do it every few minutes until the fever goes down. The boys can help you. Don't massage any place else. I can't get home before late tomorrow, but Betty is O.K. now and can take care of the baby. Bye-bye!'

"The boys did help and we rubbed that little spot in the center of Sally's toes and thumbs every few minutes all night long. It was breaking dawn when the fever went down to near normal. The next morning when Dr. H. came by to check on Sally, he was amazed at her quick recovery. 'She really had me worried,' he said. We told him what Sally had told us to do, he shook his head sadly and said, 'Too bad more people don't know how to use it; would save me a lot of work and many families a lot of heartache.' "

How a Bronchial Cough Was Stopped

A patient with a bronchial cough, under my instruction, relieved herself by pressures made with the fingers and thumb held over the bridge of her nose, and by wearing rubber bands around the thumbs and the first fingers of both hands.

This lady reported the following morning that she had enjoyed the first night's sleep she had had in more than five nights, and that a persistent and annoying headache had also cleared up.

These results are quite uniform and can be duplicated by anyone. Indeed this procedure is so simple that I have repeatedly seen bronchial and other coughs resulting from irritation or congestion at some point in the air passages, completely cured, merely by pressure on the tongue with the handle of a tablespoon or tooth brush, and many of these had persisted for a long time.

Don't underestimate the wonders of reflexology in any field of healing! If medical doctors have used and praised it so highly, then you can be thankful that the knowledge of this tremendous field of natural healing has been revealed to you.

31

How to Help Hay Fever, Asthma, and Emphysema

All sufferers from hay fever and asthma will want to read this chapter carefully. I know what it is to sneeze one's head off and then keep on sneezing and sneezing with never an end in sight. Instead of a handkerchief, I used a sheet. Sometimes I sneezed until I nearly passed out. One day I even set the house on fire because I couldn't see where I put the match after lighting the stove. I was so weak I had fallen down on the bed exhausted. I kept hearing something so I forced myself to go see what it was and there was the kitchen wall in flames. I quickly threw water on it in time to put it out. So you can see why I am in sympathy with all hay fever sufferers. And I was fast becoming a victim of asthma as well.

HELPING HAY FEVER WITH REFLEXOLOGY

Yes, Reflexology has a special message for hay fever sufferers, and this also holds true for any kind of distress in the respiratory track. The systems will all show improvement under the application of reflex message.

How a Child Was Cured of Hay Fever and Asthma

When my husband's 11-year-old daughter from a distant state came to live with us, she was suffering from hay fever and asthma. We were up with her all of the first night. The reflexes in her hands and feet were too tender for me to work on, and since she didn't know what Reflex massage was, it upset her more for me to try at that time.

She told us she had been suffering from this chronic disease for five years.

After I explained to her what Reflexology was and how it would put an end to her hay fever and asthma attacks, she gladly let me give her a treatment the next day. I started out very gently and worked only a few minutes on her that day, and to our great relief she slept soundly throughout the night.

I kept up the treatments, increasing the pressure and the time of massage every day. I also started her on raw honey and honey caps which are excellent for hay fever and asthma, and was careful of her diet. In less then three weeks, she was completely free of all signs of hay fever and asthma and has not had a sign of this distressing disease in 12 years.

HOW TO MASSAGE FOR RESPIRATORY PROBLEMS

First let us look at the fingers. We will follow the same procedure that we used for coughs and colds.

In Chart #1, you will see how the middle meridian line 1 runs down the middle of the head, through the nose and on down through the throat ending on the tips of the thumb and the big toe. Then on each side of line 1 we have line 2 which also runs down the center of the body but a little to each side, and ending in the tip of fingers number 2 and toes number 2, and the same with line 3.

By using this chart, you can understand better why the reflexes in the tongue and the first three fingers will affect the throat area.

Take the thumb in the opposite hand and massage it using the thumb and fingers all over it, searching for tender spots. When you find one then you know you are contacting a point of congestion in that area. So, remember—our motto *If it is sore, WORK IT OUT.* Massage it for a few minutes and go on searching out tender reflexes. If you find the fingers are not strong enough or get tired, the reflex comb also is helpful here. Don't forget to press the thumb on the inside next to the first finger as we did in treating coughs. After massaging the thumb, go on to the first finger and go over it with the press and massage motion searching out any tender spots, covering the finger on all sides and at the base where it is connected to the hand. Now do the same with the third or middle finger. Also massage the web between the thumb and finger and the web between the first and second fingers. Now change hands and go over the other hand in the same manner, searching for tender reflex buttons. As shown in Figure 6 in the front of the book, pressure exerted with the finger and thumb over the joints of the thumb and first and second fingers or toes has given excellent results.

Next let us use the pressure method. Keeping a steady pressure over the reflexes will achieve wonderful results. We will use a moderately tight rubber band upon the thumb and first and second fingers for ten or 15 minutes, or less if the fingers start to turn blue. If you have the reflex clamps, they will answer the same purpose without the disadvantage of having to keep a close watch for blue fingers. This is to be repeated several times a day. In fact, some of the physicians reported that they got their very best results by having their patients wear the bands as continuously as possible, removing them only long enough to allow the blood to circulate and then replacing them again. The reflex clamps can be worn continuously. These pressures exerted over the thumb and first two fingers or the toes give excellent results.

You may also use the reflex comb to exert pressure for three or four minutes at intervals, by pressing the teeth on all surfaces of the thumb and first finger, and repeating the treatment several times daily.

Use of Tongue Probe Helpful

Now let us look once again at the tongue probe. It will be used in the same manner that we used it for colds and coughs. You will press down on handle of a spoon or a knife. Do not use a sharp knife as it might slip and cut. Use the tongue probe if you have one.

The treatment of asthma and other infections of the respiratory passages is very similar to the above-mentioned methods.

Since we know that hay fever is caused by an allergy, then we will also treat the whole body to eliminate the underlying cause from malfunctioning glands and organs, especially the Ileocecal Valve (see Chart #2). Lack of calcium is one of the main reasons for allergies of all kinds, according to Doctor Smith, D. C., of Roseburg, Oregon, a good friend of mine.

How Reflexology Cures Bronchial Asthma

"Some of the cures of asthma have been little short of miraculous," says Dr. Bowers. "One patient suffering with bronchial asthma had been unable to lie down for three years; what little sleep she got was when she was propped up in a chair. Her sole relief consisted in the hypodermic injection of adrenalin solution, practically every morning and night. I made pressure on the tongue with the probe and also on the floor of the mouth directly beneath the root of the tongue.

"Within five minutes this lady—for the first time in three years—was relieved of all pain, tightness, hoarseness, and shortness of breath. In two months of this treatment, she gained 15 pounds and now sleeps through the night, and she has been able to discontinue completely her use of adrenalin.

Man Reopens Business after Reflexology
Cures Asthma

"Another bronchial asthmatic suffered so severely that he had made all arrangements to retire from business and seek health on the Riviera or in Egypt. His wheezing was so pronounced that he could be heard clear across a 20-foot room. He was advised by Dr. D. F. Sullivan, Senior Surgeon of St. Francis Hospital, to see me before leaving the country.

"I pressed on the floor of the patient's mouth, under the root of the tongue, with a probe and also made strong pressure on the first and second zones of the tongue. In three to four treatments, this man was entirely well, and informed us that he was postponing his trip abroad, and was going back into business again."

HELP FOR TUBERCULOSIS AND EMPHYSEMA
WITH REFLEXOLOGY

Since these are both deteriorating diseases of the respiratory channels, you should treat them in a similar manner when helping nature in her efforts to reactivate the cells back into a healthy condition.

You will, of course, concentrate on the reflexes to the lung which is infected, but not neglecting reflexes to the other lung. All of the reflexes in the fingers should be massaged on the sides as well as the back and palm side. Using a pressing and rolling motion, cover all fingers in this manner, also pinching and massaging the webs between the fingers. After the first two weeks you may massage the fingers in this way as often as you feel like doing it.

To help nature heal this distressing disease, you will want to stimulate the whole body, so work on all of the reflexes in both hands.

The thumb is pressed into the pad lying under the fingers which is the reflex to the lungs, as explained on page 105. Use the pressing rolling motion as you massage along this whole area. Now using the same method, work your thumb over the rest of the hand being sure to cover all of the reflexes, even those extending down into the wrists. If your thumbs and fingers are weak or become tired too quickly, you can make good use of the Magic Massager to help you stimulate the healing forces of nature by reviving electrical activity into all parts of your body. Remember in any deteriorating disease every cell in your body needs to be brought back up to perfection, not just the part that is in malfunction.

Remember to use a steady pressure to anesthetize or deaden pain, and the rotating massage to stimulate and heal.

Emphysema Victim Takes First
Deep Breath in 20 Years

Mrs. D. came to me several years ago suffering from an ailment that the doctors could give no name. She was a very sick woman with no hope of ever recovering when she walked into my office. "I know you can not help me," she said, "but to please my neighbors and my husband I am here." As I went over the reflexes, I found all of them extremely tender; her whole body was out of harmony, every gland and organ was in discord. Her hands and feet were like ice, but as I massaged them they started to get warm and pink. Mrs. D. was amazed. Even though the treatment was very painful, she did not want me to quit massaging. She said she felt as if she were coming alive all over. Because Mrs. D. had such a quick and miraculous recovery from her reflex treatments, she wanted to learn how to give these treatments to help others back to health, so I suggested she take the correspondence course, which she did.

Recently, Mrs. D. came to see me telling of the wonderful success she is having in applying this healing treatment on her friends and relatives.

"Nearly every one laughs when I mention Reflexology, but they consent to a treatment with doubts." Then, she says, "they are quite surprised at the results.

"I gave a treatment to my 77-year-old uncle who has had emphysema for years and can hardly breathe. After the treatment, he was able to take his first deep breath in 20 years."

32

How Reflexology Helps the Teeth

Is there a more unbearable pain than a toothache? And it usually strikes in the middle of the night or on a week-end when you can't get to a dentist. Or he is too busy to take you in his office for a few days, or weeks. This is where Reflexology comes to the rescue. When in pain from an aching tooth, you would do most anything to stop it. But, what to do is the question?

How to Stop an Aching Tooth with Reflexology

If the aching tooth is a front tooth on the left side, then you can see in Chart #1 how the lines from the thumb and the first finger on the left hand go down through the tooth. So you should start working on the thumb and first finger to deaden the pain. If the tooth is aching on the right side and is a back tooth, then you should look to Chart #1 and follow the lines running down the right side from fingers three, four, and five, according to where the aching tooth is located.

Use of Devices to Exert Pressure on Reflexes to Teeth

After locating the approximate area of the aching tooth, you will start to massage the reflex in the fingers lying in the correct zone lines. If the tooth is aching badly, just put pressure on these reflexes, using a comb, a clothespin, rubber bands, or even dig your fingernails in. I have known people to even use the front teeth to hold pressure on the reflexes in the fingers until the pain subsided. If you have the reflex clamps, you can use them successfully.

When the pain has subsided, you can take time to search on the fingers and even the toes for definite sore spots which will indicate the exact reflex to massage, or hold with pressure, until you can get to a dentist. You will find that this will anesthetize any area that is on the meridian line running from finger to toe.

Pressure should be made anywhere from three minutes up to 20 minutes. In one case where the patient had suffered all night, ten minutes' pressure on both sides of the fingers was used and all pains immediately stopped. Anesthesia will last from 20 minutes to three-quarters of an hour. Rubber bands on the appropriate finger or fingers seem to maintain a good effect, but you cannot leave them on for more than a few minutes at a time. You must remove them as soon as the fingers start to turn blue. The reflex clamps work well as they do not stop all of the blood circulation, which is the case when using the rubber bands. Combs may also be used by pressing the teeth into the ends of fingers.

Stops Toothache Permanently with Reflexology

I have stopped many cases of toothache by searching out tender spots on the toes and fingers, then massaging them until the pain stopped. To my surprise, several of the patients' teeth seemed to get well without the assistance of a dentist.

Now modern dentists tell us that it is possible for teeth to grow back to health if given a chance. Lennart Krook, D.V.M., Ph. D., and Leo Lutwak, Ph. D., M.D., of Cornell University, tell of carrying out a study of 80 people ranging in age from 21 to 68, who were given calcium supplementation over a period of a year which resulted in significant increases in bone density in the jaw.

Another dentist tells of treating his patients with calcium and relieving them of all types of tooth diseases. The teeth actually healed themselves when nature was called in to do her work.

Now we can easily understand how reflexology does help stop tooth problems permanently in so many cases. With a little knowledge of the tooth and its needs, you may be able to keep your teeth for as long as you live.

How a Doctor Cures Sore Teeth with Reflexology

Dr. Roemer reports a case of a man suffering from teeth so sore that he could not close his mouth. A dentist told him he could do nothing for him, so the patient had reluctantly come to him at the advice of the dentist. "I found sore spots on the inside of the thumb and first finger and made pressure on them with a comb," he goes on to tell us. "In about 5 or 6 minutes, I had him talking about his business, I asked him how his teeth were?" He was surprised to find most of the pain gone. "What did you do?" he asked. I showed him how to apply the rubber bands to his fingers and also how to use the comb to give him lasting relief from any further pain. A more thankful and grateful patient I have rarely seen, thanks to Dr. Fitzgerald's discovery of Zone Therapy (Reflexology)."

33

Treating the Eyes with Reflexology at Home

If the nerves are fatigued, the muscles of the eyes function imperfectly, as eye strain and tired muscles are largely under the control of the nervous system. Almost instant relief may be obtained by pressing the reflexes on No. 2 and No. 3 fingers and holding the pressure for several minutes.

In treating eye weaknesses, there are several things to keep in mind, but give special attention to reflexes which might be involved in any of the following: blocked circulation to the eyes caused by tight muscles in the neck due to vertebra out of alignment; faulty kidneys; diabetes; or possibly other malfunctioning glands. So, when trying to overcome any type of eye trouble, be sure to check these reflexes, giving special attention to those mentioned above and consult an eye specialist.

How to Locate Reflexes for the Eyes

For eye weaknesses, massage or press deep into the eye reflexes shown in Figure 8 in the front of the book, and note on Chart #2 how the location of the eye reflexes are located just below fingers 2 and 3. Chart #1 shows how the zone line runs from fingers 2 and 3 down through the eyes. You can also help strengthen the eyes by using pressure on the ends of these two fingers, remembering that if just one eye is involved, you will massage the reflexes on the hand and fingers on the same side as the weak eye is located. Right eye, right hand; left eye, left hand. (Figure 13 in the front of the book.)

It may be helpful if you use the reflex clamps or rubber bands to hold a steady pressure on the ends of the fingers, or the teeth of the reflex comb may be pressed into the tips of the fingers to help manifest the vital life pulsations into the eye region, thus helping nature clear out any congestion which may be causing malfunction of some part of the delicate eye canals.

The reflexes in the thumb may also be involved, so search for tender spots in all of this area of the hand, including all the webs between the fingers.

How to Relieve Eye Strain

You will find that pressure on the lower and upper side of Fingers #2 and #3 will relieve eye strain in a few minutes. You should use the finger clamps or rubber bands on these fingers five or ten minutes twice a day. Don't leave rubber bands on too long.

How to Stimulate Reflexes Around the Eyes

You will find some very sensitive reflexes around the eyes which you should also use if you are having eye problems. These reflexes will be easy to find by the tenderness as you press on the right buttons.

Hold a steady pressure and do not press too hard, *and do not use any sharp object* as it might slip and injure the eye. These reflexes cannot be reached with the fingers, so some type of smooth, solid device will have to be used such as the Reflex Hand Massager, the tongue probe, the edge of the reflex comb, or an eraser on a pencil will do. Always sterilize any object used near your eyes.

Massaging the Eye Reflexes

On the *outer edge* of your eye, which will be on meridian line 3 or 4 (Chart #1), you will feel where the bone circles the eye. Now take your device and gently press on the curve of this bone and feel for a sore reflex spot in this area, which will probably be right at the corner of the eye.

Now, using the same method, press on the bony area as it curves over the top of the eye. Search out the sore spots just as you would for a tender button in the fingers and hands.

Do the same on the under side of the eye, being sure to press on the bony structure only.

On the *inner corner* of your eye, next to the nose, you will find another tender reflex button to press. In fact, you may find several tender spots in this area along the nose.

The main button should be located right in the corner of the eye, and you will probably find it quite painful at first. There is no need for heavy pressure in these areas, so be *very gentle* with this eye massage especially.

Remember, you are not to press *into* the eye, but on the bony structure surrounding it, using a careful, steady pressure or a very light rotating massage, whichever seems to be best for your particular need.

Caution: Do not use this massage on the eye reflexes more than a few seconds, and never more than once a day for the first week or two, as these reflexes are quite powerful and might result in a headache.

Keep this work up and it will eventually eliminate your eye troubles. Remember that your body has been years running down, so don't expect to build it up in a day.

How to Use Reflexology to Stop Itching Eyes

Use the same pressure on the first, second and third fingers to help clear up sties, burning of the eyes, inflammatory conditions, and the irritating condition of granulated lids. These conditions are completely relieved when pressure is exerted on the reflexes in the fingers.

Sties are frequently relieved in one or two treatments while other conditions may take longer.

Optic Nerve Helped with Reflexology

Inflammation of the optic nerve (optic neuritis) can be very painful and lead to danger of losing the sight. Yet, this condition has been cured, as reported by one doctor, by making pressure over the first and second fingers.

Use Reflexology for Watery Eyes

To reach the tear duct of the eyes, press on the webs of the hands between the second and third fingers. You may also use a comb or other blunt device, and push upward on the lower knuckle joint of the first finger to help watering eyes. Hold until weeping stops.

Cataracts Helped with Reflex Massage

I have had success in treating cataracts with reflex massage on the feet alone. By using the above methods of reflex massage, you, too, will get wonderful results and help bring health and sparkle back into your precious eyes.

How Eye Strain Was Relieved by Reflexology

"I want you to know that my health has greatly improved and I feel like a new person since practicing the suggestions outlined in your book, 'Helping Yourself With Foot Reflexology.'

"Over the years the doctors have treated me for an enlarged heart, an over-active thyroid, impaired hearing, some arthritis in the fingers, and hemorrhoids. Three years ago I started with chiropractic treatments and found great relief. Now I am convinced that by following the methods outlined in your marvelous book, that all my discomforts will be eliminated.

"Just a few days after receiving your book, I awoke one morning to find that I was unable to read the newspaper or other fine print. This was due to using my eyes for long periods of time on needlepoint work and much reading. After massaging both feet for several weeks, my vision returned to normal.

"Thank you for compiling this priceless book."

Mrs. A.T.

Reflexology Helps Arrest Cataract

Mrs. A. gives the following report:

About six months ago, my niece was told she had pro-cataract condition of the right eye and thinning of the walls of both eyes. On recent checkups, there was a marked improvement and she was told not to come back for a year.

She told the doctor she had been using reflexology, and he agreed it was a good idea to continue it.

Thought you might be interested. I have been using it for two years and can't say enough praise for it.

34

How to Use Reflexology
to Help the Deaf Hear

It is hard to make people believe that by pressing on the joints of the ring, or fourth and fifth fingers or toes, that the hearing of the adjacent ear can be *benefited.* Yet this is a fact. A similar result will follow by pressing with a solid device such as an eraser on the reflex on the jaw behind the wisdom tooth.

Physicians, familiar with the practice and principles of Zone Therapy (Reflexology) have used this method and claimed that nine out of ten cases of otosclerosis (thickening of the ear membranes) can be improved up to 90 percent. It will help "ear noise"; and ringing in the ears can be helped in over 90 percent of the cases. If there is any hearing left you will almost certainly be able to improve it.

Osteopaths, chiropractors, and naturopathic doctors who have not hesitated to use this method of healing have frequently had some startling results.

One doctor tells of a dentist curing or helping more than 20 of his patients by using this simple yet beneficial treatment of reflex pressure to help the deaf hear.

You also can use this method to help bring back hearing. Use pressure on the end of the ring finger, being sure to treat the finger of the left hand if it is the left ear that is troubling you, and the right hand if it is the right ear. Treat both hands if both of your ears are not functioning as they should.

One simple way to hold this pressure is with a spring clothespin on the end of the ring finger. Another is to use a rubber band around the end of the ring finger, being sure to remove it as soon as the

185

fingers begin to turn blue. Do this several times a day until all symptoms of ear congestion, deafness, ringing in the head, etc. have disappeared. See Figure 14 in the front of the book.

Also, you can place a sterile wad of hard cotton in the space between the last tooth and the angle of the jaw. This is in back of the wisdom tooth. There is a reflex in this area that goes to the ear, and is stimulated by a steady pressure. So you bite down hard on this object for about five minutes, repeating this treatment several times a day.

Using a sterilized hard rubber eraser instead of the cotton seems to work even better, or you may find something which serves the purpose better for you.

You can also use the reflex comb to press the tips of all of the fingers thus sending the healing life force into malfunctioning ears, holding this pressure for about five minutes.

However in order to maintain hearing improvement, it is important that you be persistent with the treatments. In some cases, if treatments are discontinued for any appreciable length of time, the condition sometimes returns. So even if your hearing has returned, don't neglect to use these reflex pressures often on the so important little push buttons to the ears.

The reflex clamps work well in holding a steady pressure on the fingers when treating the ears as well as other malfunctioning parts of the body, and are not uncomfortable. See Figure 13 in the front of this book and Figure 10-2 in the chapter on clamps.

CASE HISTORIES FROM FILES OF MEDICAL DOCTORS

It does sound too simple and easy to be true, doesn't it? but let me give you a few case histories from the files of medical doctors who have used these methods with such great success. It may then be easier to put the teaching into practical use and benefit from this simple technique of massage to free yourself of all ear troubles by squeezing and pressing the fingers for a few minutes, several times a day.

Doctor's Wife Hears after 30 Years

The wife of an ear specialist was brought to me for treatment for deafness. The doctor had tried unsuccessfully every accredited method and was constrained to see what zone therapy could do.

For 30 years this patient had heard nothing with the right ear, and very little with the left. I stimulated with a curved cotton tipped probe the area lying between the last tooth and the angle of the jaw. After two treatments, this patient could hear a small tuning fork one-half inch away from the right ear, and one inch from the left. After a few treatments, her hearing so wonderfully improved that she could hear a whisper with the right ear. This, after being deaf for 30 years, and after having visited all the noted aurists in this country and abroad.

Singer Recovers Hearing

A young soprano member of a leading Hartford church choir, suffered a progressive loss of hearing, which finally became so pronounced as to make it almost impossible for her to "sing on the pitch," or harmonize with either the organ or the other quartet members.

She received treatment similar to that employed on the doctor's wife, supplementing it by "home treatment." This consisted of tucking a wad of surgeon's cotton or a solid rubber eraser in the space in back of the wisdom tooth, and having her bite forcibly upon it, repeating the procedure several times daily, especially immediately before singing or rehearsing. In a few weeks, this girl had completely recovered her hearing, and was able to accept an engagement with a traveling concert company.

The doctor reporting on her case goes on to say, "I have had to date, possibly 50 cases of deafness of one kind or another, all of whom have been helped materially."

Minister Cured from Otosclerosis in Minutes

One patient, a minister afflicted with otosclerosis for 25 years, (supposed thickening of the membranes of the inner ear), could barely hear loud talking. After working for five minutes upon the joints of the third (ring) finger, and to a lesser degree, upon its two neighbors, it was found that the patient could hear a whisper twenty feet away.

As proof of this, it was whispered to him, "Will you close the window above your head?" He arose immediately from his chair and obliged.

How Physician's Relative Regained Hearing

A New York physician had a relative who had been unsuccessfully treated for deafness in one ear (the right) by conventional methods for the past 16 years, by some of the most famous aurists in New York, London, Paris, Berlin, Dresden, Vienna, and other centers of medical learning. X-ray treatment had at one time made this case at least 25 percent worse. With the left ear, this patient could hear a loud voice "close up."

Dr. Reid Kellogg volunteered to "show the doctor something", using this case for demonstration purposes. The doctor, like Barkis, being "willing," our friend took his trusty aluminum comb from his pocket and exerted pressure for five minutes with the teeth of the comb on the tips of the patient's left hand. He also used the pressure in the mouth for an additional five minutes with a rubber eraser placed behind the wisdom tooth.

The doctor then stood ten feet away from his relative and talked to him in an ordinary tone of voice. The patient heard distinctly with the left ear every word spoken.

Our doctor then started to work on the other hand while the patient was protesting that this was a waste of time because some of the "biggest" ear specialists in Europe had failed to help the right ear. However, the attempt was made, and within ten minutes the patient heard a clock a foot away, a watch held three inches distant from his ear, and he further was able to repeat words spoken loudly two feet away. During the experiments with his right ear the left ear was tightly plugged so this test was quite conclusive.

Deaf Parents Made to Hear With Reflexology

A lady and her husband who were both deaf came to this doctor, but the baby in her arms was not deaf, and most decidedly was not dumb either. In less than a fortnight's treatment, both parents could hear the baby cry every night, which was a great satisfaction to them in one way—but they don't know yet whether to laugh or cry about it.

Have you read enough to convince you of the wonderful results of reflexology for the ears? Let me quote two more case histories.

Hearing Returned to Deaf Soldier

A veteran who had been deafened by a gun concussion was treated by using the pressure behind the teeth on the gum margins near the angle of the jaw. He was then able to hear for the first time in years. That it was a pleasure, was evidenced by the fact that the old soldier danced around the office in a perfect transport of glee.

Skeptic Cured after 39 Years of Deafness

One lady, aged 45, deaf since she was six years old, came to the office of a specialist who studied Zone Therapy (Reflexology). When the physician applied a comb to one hand, she whispered "crank" to a friend. Twenty minutes later, being able to hear ordinary conversation, she whispered "wizard."

HOW TO EASE AN ACHING EAR

We have found one of the most effective and quickest cures for an earache to be pressure exerted on the end of the fourth finger (ring finger) for about five minutes.

In case of emergency, any pressure or manipulation of this area is effective. An ordinary spring clothespin or a rubber band are handy devices to use and will bring relief from pain almost immediately. You may even use the teeth to exert pressure to stop pain by biting the end of the finger. If you have the reflex clamps they give particularly good results, with greater comfort then the aforementioned home devices.

To start the vital life forces activating the congestion which has been causing the trouble, hold a steady pressure on the tip of the ring finger of the hand which is located on the same side as the aching ear. Keep this pressure on the finger until the ear stops aching or you can get a doctor.

Deafness is seldom sudden but creeps in so subtly that we refuse to acknowledge the condition as if it were some kind of disgrace. To keep a continuous watch over its possible onset, test your hearing by listening to your watch tick. If you can't hear it, chances are you are already "hard of hearing."

How a Socialite Regained Hearing

Mrs. L.P., a rich proud socialite, was unable to tell if her expensive watch needed repairs since she could not hear its usual ticking. Only then did she realize that her hearing was at fault, even though she blamed her inability to catch other sounds to distracting noises, and occasional failure to distinguish words to poor speech. The discovery was a great shock and source of unhappiness, since she did not want to be forced to wear a hearing aid or be suspected of oncoming senility. One of her friends, who had cured her own partial deafness, told her about her own experience with Reflexology.

Mrs. L.P. took her friend's advice and immediately started using Reflexology as directed by her friend. Her hearing was soon restored to normal, thus preserving not only her health but also her vanity.

Being "hard of hearing" or totally deaf is a serious affliction, not only for the sufferer but a source of callous impatience and lack of compassion on the part of others, if not outright derision. The old-fashioned ear trumpet is still a prime source of comedy. It is no wonder that we hesitate to acknowledge its onset. Even with our advanced and modern designs of hearing aids, there are many who refuse to wear them. Now, however, thanks to the miracle healing power of Hand Reflexology, we can treat hearing loss promptly without expensive hearing aids, medication, or special equipment.

You Can Help Hearing-Loss in Children

Hearing loss in children is often overlooked, even in these modern days of testing in the schools. It has been learned that poor hearing may be the cause of poor speech since the child is unable to hear spoken words clearly, or of low grades because he is unable to hear the teacher. He needs understanding and help, not scolding or accusations. To guard your child's emotional and physical health, a simple Reflexology treatment once a week may help to insure perfect hearing in the future and a happy well adjusted life.

You can teach him to use Reflexology on himself, as most children enjoy using this natural way to help themselves maintain good health.

35

How to Cure a Sick Voice
with Reflexology

We will all agree that a sick voice is one of the most frustrating things that can happen to anyone. We don't realize how much we talk until our voice suddenly becomes silent. Sometimes people suffer for several weeks from laryngitis, barely able to speak above a whisper, not knowing that all they had to do was apply a few minutes of reflex pressure on the fingers and the tongue to get almost immediate and lasting relief.

The technique of working on the reflexes in the tongue has many benefits in certain instances which involve the area around the head and throat, as is mentioned in other chapters.

Let us first apply the finger massage, which mainly involves the thumb, and to a lesser degree, the first and second fingers. We usually work on the fingers of both hands when stimulating the areas of the throat, since the throat box is centralized and would be on the Zone 1 line with lines 2 and 3 being close to give radiations of healing to a lesser degree. See Charts #1 and #2.

Take the thumb of the left hand and press the right hand thumb along the inside of the thumb, the part which touches the index finger.

Notice in Figure 35-1 how the fingers are pressed into the inner side of the thumb which is definitely a reflex to the voice in the vocal cord zone. Keep searching in this area for a sharp sore spot, and when you find it, massage it for a few minutes, then change hands and search out the tender reflex on the opposite thumb in the same

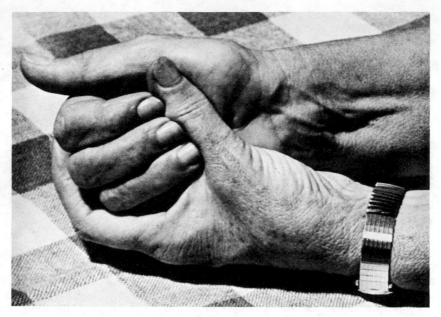

Figure 35-1. Position for pressing the inner side of thumb.

manner. Now go all over both thumbs in the same manner, massaging one thumb at a time. Also massage the webs on both hands. The reflex clamps may also be used, putting pressure on both thumbs at the same time. Rubber bands or a clothespin may be used in an emergency if you do not have the clamps.

Digging the fingernails into the reflexes on the inside of the thumb is also useful when nothing else is available.

Great Singer Uses Reflexology to Ease Throat Tension

Now we come to the technique of stimulating the reflexes in the tongue. As explained in another chapter, you will take a clean cloth and place it around the tongue; now take it between the thumb and fingers and gently pull it out as far as comfortable, then wiggle it from side to side. This will relieve a "tight," inflexible throat, which is the bane of all vocalists and speakers. This method, for instance, was used for many years by the gifted Italian tenor, Umberto Sorrentino. He says, "This method eases up throat tension, and frees the voice, and will abort a cold."

Reflexology Used by Opera Singer to Keep Voice Beautiful

Miss Mabel Garrison, a lyric soprano of the Metropolitan Opera House, also used this method of reflexology not only on herself, but has won the appreciation and gratitude of various members of the company, by curing their stiff, inelastic sore throats.

It is a significant fact that no singer, lawyer, actor, clergyman, mother of a family, or businessman can afford to ignore the simple application of reflexology when the voice is affected.

Grandmothers Used Reflexology to Relieve Choking in Croup

Another procedure which can help ease an ailing voice is the probe method on the reflexes in the tongue. In case of coughing and choking as in croup, our grandmothers knew how to relieve this distress by placing the finger on the back of the tongue and pressing it for a few minutes until the coughing stopped.

Many Speakers Turn to Reflexology for Relief of Vocal Strain

Reflexology has, in innumerable instances, restored lost speaking voices. It is a common occurrence to have a clergyman, a lawyer, and other businessmen who have become voiceless from long dictation, or some other vocal strain go to a reflexologist, unable to speak above a whisper, and within a half hour go their way rejoicing.

How a Speaker Regained His Voice

It is remarkable what the finger pressures alone will accomplish. Mr. A., a politician, had been speaking most of the day at a convention held in a grove. The amplifier refused to work so he talked without it. The leafy bowers and mossy dells were not built for acoustic purposes and the consequence was that when darkness closed in Mr. A. could not speak above a whisper. He had such a contraction of the muscles that he couldn't even open his jaws—let alone talk through them.

When he presented himself at the office of a reflexologist the next day, he could not open his mouth. It was impossible to treat the reflexes in the tongue, so he was given an aluminum comb and told to press the teeth on the reflexes on the hands, starting with the end of the thumb and working down to the wrist; also around the first and second fingers covering the whole area, pressing both on the palm and the back side of the hand, including the webs. He was left to his own devices for about 20 minutes. At the end of this time, the tension of the jaw muscles had relaxed, and he had also relieved the irritation in his throat. A tongue depressor was then used, and three days later he was able to resume his speaking.

Technique of Finding Reflexes in the Tongue

To use this same technique it is better to use the clean handle of a table knife, or a spoon handle if you do not have a tongue probe, to press down on the reflexes on the back of the tongue. In case of emergency, the finger can be used, of course. Just place whatever device is being used in the back part of the mouth without making yourself gag, and press down on the tongue, searching for tender spots here as you would on the fingers. When you find a tender spot hold the pressure on it for a few seconds or minutes, according to the condition of your throat. Sterilize any object before putting it into the mouth.

Almost everyone suffers occasionally from defects somewhere in the delicate mechanism that shapes the air currents into beautiful sounds, and molds the breath into speech.

Professional Performers Helped by Reflexology

In other arts such as ballet, theater, etc., where performers must remain at the peak of talent at all times, reflexology treatments have helped in many ways: better breath control, fewer colds, relaxation from tension both muscular and of the nervous system which are a threat to performance, all of which resulted in greater confidence and less anxiety. An important voice teacher in the city often sent students to Reflexologist Mrs. Roon, to give help in these areas.

Mrs. Roon had been a professional singer herself and understood well what the problems could be and how to help them with Reflex Massage. She was a dear person, full of projects and activities and always glad to be of help.

How to Relax While Making a Speech

My son-in-law tells me of an experience he had with Reflexology without realizing what he was doing.

He had to give a talk to a group of salesmen and not being used to making speeches, he was quite nervous. He said he was so upset when he first got up in front of the group that he couldn't even think of the lines he had practiced beforehand. In his nervousness, he unconsciously pressed the tips of his fingers together as he talked, and suddenly he felt relaxed and at ease as he continued his talk, finishing it with great success. But he remembers that he kept the tips of his fingers pressed tightly together all through the talk.

Now he realizes that it was the act of pressing the fingers together which brought him relaxation at the high point of tension and made it possible to feel at ease through the rest of his speech. But at the time he was not aware of using one of nature's powerful forces to relaxing his nerves.

Press the tips of all your fingers together as in Figure 4 in the front of the book, with a slight pressure for a few moments and feel the surge of electric currents vibrating through your body.

36

How to Stop Falling Hair with Reflexology

A beautiful frame brings to life even the dullest of pictures.

Your hair is the frame for your face and its beauty or lack of beauty makes the difference in how you look to the world. Baldness used to confine itself mostly to men, but today women put their hair under so much stress from the use of chemicals for permanents, dyes, etc. that they are taking their place along with the balding men.

Hair Is Barometer of Your Health

Hair, like the nails, is a modified skin structure similar to the outer layer of the skin. The hair is peculiarly sensitive to the condition of the health of the body. If, for any cause, the system is depleted, it shows in the hair before any other place.

Scientists tell us to take protein for beautiful hair and strong, beautiful fingernails; yet, no one has mentioned the vital electrical force activating stimulation between the hair and nails. Both the hair and nails are made of the same substance and are cut at regular intervals. They are on the same electrical current of healing forces waiting for the right button to be pushed to help nature revive glandular activity.

Doctor Gives Magic Secret of How to Grow New Hair

I am going to tell you the secret, told by the late Dr. Joe Shelby Riley, that will not only stop your falling hair, but will help you grow a new head of hair successfully. If you are combing your hair out by the handfuls, then you will be forever grateful for yet another of nature's simple techniques of using reflexology not only to free you from the embarrassment of falling hair, but also to help you grow a beautiful new head of hair though you are now bald. HERE IS THE MAGIC SECRET:

Rub the fingernails of one hand directly across the fingernails of the other hand with a quick, rapid motion as though you were buffing them with a buffer, only you are using the fingernails of the opposite hand as the buffer. Do this for five minutes at least three times a day. (See Figure 16 in the front of the book.)

How to Use Reflexology to Prevent Gray Hair

This miracle of new hair won't happen in a day or two. You must keep at it. The first thing you will notice in a few weeks is that the hair has stopped falling out. If you are young, that is, before your hair has begun to turn gray, and you do this for five minutes night and morning, you will build up the entire nerve force of your body. As nerve force is the foundation of a perfect organ, stimulate the hair molecules into life and you will have plenty of hair as long as you live and will never have a gray hair the rest of your life. We cannot, of course, give you examples of this, but can only say that thousands of people, 60 and 70 years of age who have been doing this all their lives, are living witness to the truth of this statement. Concentrate on this as you do it. Don't let up. Keep in mind what you wish to accomplish.

This magic secret of stimulating the reflexes in the fingernails will be a boon, not only to balding men, but especially to women who have discovered that first gray hair.

Previously Bald Author Has Luxurious Hair at 70

The author of this system was bald and said, as many others have said,

Oh, it is natural to be bald. My father was bald and my grandfather was bald before he was forty. I quit wearing a hat and started to use the exercises as described above, and soon my head began to have a fuzz, and then the hair began to grow, and now at over 70 years of age I have a fine luxurious head of hair.

Many thousands who have used this natural method of reflex massage now rejoice because of the beautiful head of hair that frames their faces.

I repeat Dr. Riley's statement: *Go Thou and Do Likewise.*

"GIVE NATURE A CHANCE."

37

Using Reflexology to Treat "Female Weaknesses" and Sex Glands

The reproduction organs are the strongest part of any species. I don't know of any part of the body that can cause more suffering and unhappiness over a long period of time than malfunctioning reproductive organs. When these organs are out of tune, then truly the whole system is rasping in disharmony.

I suffered from my first period. Every month, I went through an agony of pain equal to labor pains although I did not know this until I married and my first baby was born. The doctor was in a hurry to go home, so he took the baby with instruments and pulled my uterus loose from the muscles. This caused a constant feeling of discomfort in the lower region of my body from the navel down. Anyone having trouble in the reproductive organs knows the feeling, everything hurts! Two years later, I had another baby with no trouble, and a few months later, the doctor operated and tied my uterus back into place.

Not long after this, I started having cysts on the cervix and would have to have them burned off every few months. I was not the only one that suffered in the ensuing years. I could not be a normal wife or mother because I always had a dull, heavy feeling from the waist down. I was nervous and irritable. I was lucky to have a kind and understanding husband.

After we moved to Idaho, I had a bad spell and went to a doctor there who hurt me on examining me. He told me that I had cancer, and that he had to operate immediately. I knew this was not true as I had just been to my own doctor before leaving California.

How Old-Fashioned Doctor Ends Cyst Troubles

I then went to another old-time doctor. His office looked clean, but old-dated. When I told him my problems of many years' standing, he was furious, not at me, but at doctors. He said, "There is no reason in the world why any woman should have female troubles. The reproductive organs are the easiest to heal in the whole body because nature set them up to reproduce. They respond to the simplest of treatment." He cauterized the cyst and gave me a prescription. "You take this tonic and you will never have any more trouble." I asked him if I could have another baby and he said I was too scarred by cysts to carry one if I ever did get pregnant. Well, I did get pregnant one month after taking the tonic and had a perfect baby girl.

We went back to California in a few months and I went into a drugstore to have the prescription filled. The druggist said he would send on to the doctor in Idaho for it. I waited for weeks and he kept saying it hadn't come in yet. One day, I got mad and told him I wanted it, so he said, "Oh, yes, we got it, but it called for some old-fashioned ingredients. We don't use the "L.P." stuff anymore. I told him what I thought—that if they used it, there would be no more drugs to sell to suffering women, and no more operations for the doctors to perform. He just laughed.

Reflexology and Tonic Ends Operations

I got along fine for several years after my baby was born. One day, I had pains in the lower part of my body. I went to my doctor and he said, "cysts again", and I had to be cauterized once more. I thought, "Oh, no, here we go again." Then I remembered that wonderful old-fashioned doctor in Idaho. I went to the drugstore and bought a bottle of the "old-fashioned" patent medicine ("Lydia Pinkham") and I have never had trouble again. That was 20 years ago, and I have never been to a doctor since for female weaknesses. Of course, I then learned the technique of reflexology and never had to worry anymore, but I still keep a bottle of the L.P. "tonic" on my shelf. I used it for my daughters through their adolescent years. Even today, if they mention troubles in the region of the reproductive organs, I tell them to massage their reflexes and take some L.P. tonic.

I tell you this story to let you know the needlessness of suffering from any kind of female disorders. The reproductive organs will heal themselves when nature is given a chance.

IMPORTANCE OF SEX GLANDS

The reflexes of the gonads or sex glands in both male and female are of the utmost importance, not only in helping nature stimulate these reproductive organs and glands back to life if they are in a state of malfunction, but also to keep them in perfect order for the welfare of your whole system.

The testes of men and the ovaries of women are associated almost exclusively with their reproductive functions. While reproduction is unquestionably the most important function of the gonads, the hormones which they produce have far-reaching effects on the body generally, and even upon mental activity.

Certain distinct cells of the ovaries and the testes devote themselves to the production of steroid hormones, while others evolve into spermatozoa and ova. Both functions are closely related to and controlled by the pituitary gland.

In Chart #3 on Endocrine Glands in the beginning of the book, you will see the position of the sex glands and organs. Then look at Chart #2 and you will see the position of the corresponding reflexes.

How to Help Prostate, Penis, and Uterus with Reflexology

Congestion of the prostate gland, also the penis and uterus, can be helped by using reflex massage on the entire lower lumbar area. You can see in Figure 37-1, how the thumb of one hand is placed on the reflexes on the wrist lying just below the thumb on the opposite hand. In your Chart #2, you can find the location of these organs and also see how the meridian Zone Lines on Chart #1 run from fingers one and two down through this area to the toes; also how they pass through the pituitary gland located in the head.

To help stimulate these glands with the healing forces of nature, massage not only the reflexes that directly correspond to the above mentioned glands, but also the endocrine glands as well since they

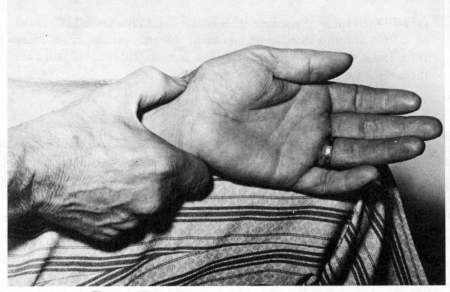

Figure 37-1. Position for massaging the reflexes to the prostate, uterus, and penis.

are all interrelated. You can see how pressure and massage on the thumb and the first finger will affect all the glands and organs involved. The tongue probe will also be of much help when there is malfunction of any kind in this area. The whole lumbar area should be stimulated by using the massage of the wrists, the clamps on the fingers, and even the Magic Massager can help here since it will give added benefits by massaging all of the other glands to create harmony and stimulate an added glandular activity in the whole system.

Since nature saw fit to move the reflexes of these most important glands from the bottom of the feet up to the ankles (probably so they would not become over-stimulated as they were walked on), she may have moved the gonad reflexes to the wrists of the hands for the same reason.

You will find the reflexes in this area of the wrist to the ovaries, uterus, and fallopian tubes in the female; and the testicles, penis, and prostate glands in the male.

Look at the Zone Chart #1 and notice how the meridian Line

No. 1 runs down through the center of the penis, prostate and the uterus, while Lines No. 2 and No. 3 run through the ovaries and the testes. You can see how the pituitary gland influences these organs in the center of the body, while the pineal, thyroid, and adrenals carry their influence to the ovaries and testes.

Technique

Note the position of the thumb on the wrist in Figure 37-1. To massage the reflexes for congestion or malfunction of the prostate and the penis in the male and the uterus in the female, place the thumb of one hand on the spot a little below the base of the thumb of the opposite hand. Now, with a pressing, rolling motion, massage this whole area, searching for a tender spot. When you find it, you will know you are on the right button. Keep massaging for a few minutes, then change hands and massage the reflex on the other wrist. Don't be surprised if you find one side more tender than the other as often happens.

Pituitary

By studying Chart #2 and the Zone Chart #1, we see that the thumbs of both hands should also be massaged to stimulate the pituitary gland. Press the edge of one thumb into the center of the pad on the thumb of the opposite hand, giving it a deep massage to help stimulate the vital life force back into the channels which are in relation to the above organs.

How to Quiet Pain with Reflexology

Remember, to stimulate and heal, we use an agitating motion of massage; to quiet down or deaden pain, we use pressure. If you are trying to stop pain, then it will be better for you to put pressure on the thumb. Since the gonads, or sex glands, are lower down in the body, you might have more success by applying the pressure near the base of the thumb. If you use rubber bands or clamps, place them as close to the hand as possible. Use your fingers to search out tender spots on the thumb and when you find them, hold a steady pressure for about 15 minutes at a time.

Thyroid or Adrenals, Ovaries, and Testes

Now, let us turn to the reflexes to the ovaries and testes which are on Zone Lines No. 2 and No. 3. If there is a malfunction here, as stated above, we should work on the reflexes to the thyroid and the adrenals. Since these are on both sides of the body, massage the reflexes in both hands, concentrating on the side which is affected most.

Look at Figure 37-2 and see how the thumb is placed on the wrist under the same side as the little finger is on. Massage this area much the same as you did for the penis, prostate, and the uterus. Massage the first and second fingers or use pressure on them if there is pain as you did on the thumbs.

Have you noticed that these are all of the endocrine group? Besides massaging fingers No. 1 and No. 2, you will massage the thyroid reflex under the base of the thumb as shown in Figure 5 in

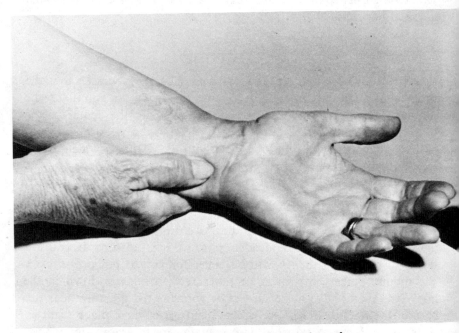

Figure 37-2.   Position for massaging the reflexes to the ovaries and the testes.

the front of the book and explained in the chapter on thyroid, and also the adrenal glands which should be given special attention when there is trouble in this region of the body.

Notice how the thumb is placed on the center of the hand in Figure 7 in the front of the book, to massage the adrenals. Also notice how the other reflexes are crowded together here, so when one of these reflexes is massaged, the others also get their share of stimulation. The Magic Massager will work well in massaging these reflexes which are in relation to the sex gland area.

SEX GLANDS OF MEN AND WOMEN

Both men and women who have suffered from malfunctioning of the sex glands know how the whole lower part of the body is affected. It feels as if infection has set in from the waist down, so let us massage all of this lower lumbar area for relief. Massage all of the wrist, working the fingers clear across from side to side and even on up the wrist a ways if it feels tender. The Rollo Massager is helpful here. (See Figure 37-3.)

Reflexes in Tongue Relieve Weakness of Sex Glands

Now we will go on to the value and technique of pressing the reflexes in the tongue. This seems to be the most potent reflex area in controlling pain and malfunctioning of the reproductive organs.

The success and validity of this method of treatment is told by several doctors; I will give you their versions and some of their case histories.

In the chapter on the reflexes in the tongue, you were hold how to use the tongue probe for various situations.

Let us see how this method was successfully put to use by such doctors as Wm. Fitzgerald, M.D., George White, M.D., Edwin F. Bowers, M.D., etc. There were many others who used this method with great enthusiasm at the amazing results they were getting in helping their patients.

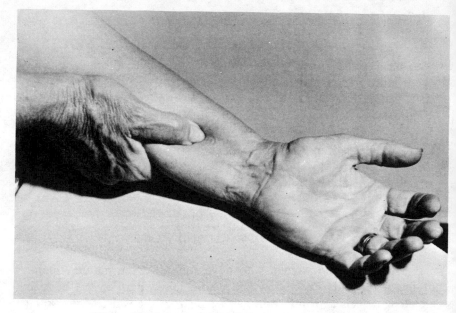

Figure 37-3. Position for massaging reflexes.
to the lower lumbar area.

How Reflex Pressure Started a Girl's Period
in Five Minutes

"Many of the things Zone Therapy (Reflexology) does are positively startling. And yet they become commonplace after one has been in the work for a time," says Dr. White. I agree with him one hundred percent.

How Painless Menstration Is Started in Five Minutes

One of the most striking cases that has yet come to my attention came in the form of a letter of thanks from the mother of a young girl. The mother said that her daughter had not menstruated in ten months. She was instructed by a former patient of mine to take the broad handle of a tablespoon and make strong pressure on the tongue as far back as she could stand it without gagging. She did so and within five minutes she was menstruating profusely, yet without the slightest pain or discomfort. In the several months following, she had her period regularly every 28 days. The mother, who had feared her daughter was going into a "decline", could not refrain from writing me a most heartfelt letter of appreciation for what my former patient had been able to do for her daughter. I call this good preventive medicine.

Painful Menstruation Is Also Helped

By using the probe on the tongue, you can control the painful hours of menstruation like magic. No longer will you need the deadening influence of drugs You can relieve the pain in the back and thighs, as well as other menstrual complaints, by the simple method of holding pressure with the handle of a large spoon pressed down on the back of the tongue. This should be applied to the tongue three-quarters of the way back.

The pressure should be held firmly for two or three minutes and then relaxed, and the point of pressure changed slightly to one side and then the other side. Keep in mind that you are pressing on the meridian line No. 1 in the center and when you move the probe over slightly, you will be on line No. 2 or No. 3. Remember, these are the zones which affect the sex organs in which you are activating the healing forces of nature. Women have taken to carrying the tongue probe in their purse to relieve monthly complaints.

Many women who had to take to their beds for two or three days each month or use a series of drugs, are now finding relief of all distress after a course in this treatment. Most of them say they hardly know when their period starts. Don't forget, pressure on the thumbs and the first two fingers can be used in conjunction with the tongue probe technique.

Profuse Menstruation Slowed with Comb Technique

If there is a too-profuse and too-frequent menstruation, tongue pressures should not be used. It will be better to use the more soothing technique of combing the back of the hands with the teeth of the reflex comb, and also the quieting pressure can be used on the fingers and wrists as explained earlier in this chapter.

Warning of Miscarriage Cause

I want to sound a word of warning here, however, to anyone who is pregnant. *Do not* use the tongue depressor method as it might induce a *miscarriage,* particularly during the early months. If this tongue pressure can start the menstrual period in five minutes, then it is quite conceivable that abortion might follow drastic tongue treatment. One should also be careful about biting the tongue or holding pressure on it with the teeth while pregnant. It will be better to depend on finger pressures, during these months.

I have just given you the *magic key* with which to unlock the door that will free you from the pain and distress of being a woman, forever. All you have to do is use it. It is free!

Reflex Massage Stops Hot Flashes

Dear Mrs. Carter:

I want to tell you how much we have enjoyed your book on Reflexology, and how much good it has done. We have purchased about six books ourselves and given them away to members of our family and friends. Also we have told many of our friends about the reflex massage, and they have become interested and bought the book. I don't think there is one that it hasn't helped in one way or another.

As for myself, I began having hot flashes a few months ago and it stopped them completely. What a relief, the mysterious fainting spells also stopped.

My husband who is 70 years old was having trouble of some sort. We didn't know what. Doctors didn't seem to know either. One said he had diabetes, which it turned out he didn't have. Anyhow he was having spells where he would almost pass out several times a day. His back was pretty much out of line, which we didn't know. He had been going to a chiropractor for several years, but they couldn't seem to help much. So to make a long story short, he started with the foot reflexology. His passing-out spells stopped in about a week. He has massaged his feet for about a year now. He says he can feel the bones in his spine and neck move, and slip back and forth. He feels much better. So needless to say, he is a firm believer in reflexology.

Mrs. R.D.S.

Nun Helps Sister Nun
Back to Health with Reflexology
A Nun Reports:

I think of you every day with gratitude. A little over a week ago a young Sister friend was feeling very ill and had gone to bed. "What's the trouble?" I asked, "your period?" "No," she replied, "I wish it were." She hadn't had one for a year. So I gave her a treatment and said I'd continue to do so for a month, then if nothing happened she should see a gynecologist. Next morning she could hardly wait to tell me it had already begun. And it continued normally.

So I am giving her a treatment every night and I am praying the cycle will be normalized. You can imagine my joy since you experience it constantly yourself.

I am feeling very well, perhaps thanks to one-half hour of massaging my feet every day.

With affection and prayerful wishes.

Sister L.M.

How Prostate Is Cured Almost Immediately

Mr. A. reports: "I want to tell you how wonderful I think reflexology is. Although I am only in my early thirties, I have had prostate trouble along with other health problems for the past two years. After studying your reflexology hand charts, I decided to try it on myself. I massaged all of the reflex areas in both wrists and felt almost immediate relief.

"Then I massaged all of the reflexes in both hands. Now I am free of all prostate trouble and the rest of my illnesses seem to have vanished also, and I feel great for the first time in two years.

"Thank you for introducing me to Reflexology. From now on it will have top priority in my family."

38

Reflex Technique for Painless Childbirth

Any woman who has gone through the pangs of childbirth with or without drugs will welcome the news of a natural, painless method of delivery with no drugs or anesthetics to endanger her health and the life of her unborn infant.

Any method, no matter how improbable it sounds, is worthy of consideration by any physician, and especially, it could be a boon to those who now choose to have their babies at home, as so many women are doing today. They need only to turn to nature and the use of modern "push button" techniques to bring their babies painlessly and safely into the world. As explained below, with the help of a couple of combs a woman starting into delivery can press the teeth of the comb into the reflexes in her hands to help relax the muscles, allowing the baby to be born in a short time with very little pain, thus making the birth easy for the mother and child and giving them both a better chance for life without danger of complications setting in.

Technique: As soon as labor pains begin, the mother should be given a comb for each hand (See Figure 8-1) and something solid to press her feet against. Although ordinary household combs can be used, they are apt to break under pressure and injure the fingers. For this reason, Reflex Combs which are specially designed for the purposes of hand reflexology are recommended.

Holding the combs' teeth down, the patient exerts pressure across the tops by pressing down firmly with the fingers until the teeth dig into the palm area, as hard as can be comfortably borne and maintaining constant pressure. If the hands become tired, relax them for a few minutes, and continue the pressure. The combs should be held across the palm, or wherever it seems most comfortable to the patient. At the same time, press the soles of the feet hard against a footboard which should have a rough rather than a smooth surface.

The patient might find more relief by turning the combs upside down and pressing the teeth into the tips of the fingers and the ends of the thumbs. (See Figure 8-2.)

How Reflexology Relieves Labor Pains

In the first stage of labor, reflexology relieves the nagging pains without retarding, but rather promoting, dilation. In the second stage, delivery is hastened. This natural method of helping the mother deliver quickly and painlessly should be a great boon to doctors and nurses, and especially to the delivering mother and her baby.

Reflexology Technique Used Instinctively by Women in Labor

This method of help in time of labor is merely an amplification of techniques that have always been used instinctively by women. The clenching of the hands, the crushing grasp on the hands of the attendant, etc. are nature's own methods of bringing relief from pain in labor. They are inadequate, however, because the pressures are not maintained for a sufficient length of time and because the means for making the pressure are not sufficiently·"sharp." In other words, nature knows what should be done but she doesn't go far enough with it. Zone Therapy (Reflexology) merely increases the effectiveness of an already existing method by improving on it.

Doctor White Lectures on Easy Childbirth

In a lecture to physicians on "Easy Childbirth," Doctor White stated:

> Any method calculated to render labor less of an ordeal—particularly when the method can possibly do no harm—is worthy of trial. There is absolutely no danger to either mother or child in its employment, for in almost every case in which

Zone Therapy (Reflexology), has been tried, labor has been accelerated three hours or more, instead of retarded.

Use Comb Technique Only When Doctor Is Present

Before going on to some case histories, I want to emphasize most strongly to those readers who are expecting a baby, not to try this method by yourselves, or you might suddenly find yourself alone with a new-born baby! In these days of poor nutrition or indifference to proper diets, lack of enough exercise, etc. there could be complications, in which case you would need your doctor with you. It might mean the life of your baby or even your own, so be sure that the *doctor is available.*

I have never delivered a baby myself, but I wish I had known of this method when I had my own first baby delivered by instruments, and again when I was forced to have a Caesarean with a later child after hours of suffering.

Now I am going to give you some actual case histories taken from the files of prominent medical doctors who did use Zone Therapy (Reflexology) when natural methods of healing and doctoring were still considered in style.

Young Mother Has Painless Delivery When Doctor Uses Reflexology

Doctor R. T. H. Nesbitt of Waukegan, Illinois, gives this report on his first experience with zone pressure in a confinement case after attending a lecture by Doctor White:

"As I was expecting a confinement call every hour, I told Doctor White and he gave me some special pointers concerning this work. Last night I was called to attend what I expected would be my last case of confinement, as I have been doing this work so many years that I intended to retire. From my last night's experience, I feel as if I should like to start the practice of medicine all over again.

"The woman I delivered was a primipara (one who had never had a child before), and who, therefore, because of the rigidity of the bones and tissues, has a more difficult labor.

"When severe contractions began, and the mother was beginning to be very nervous and complained of pain, at which time I generally administer an anesthetic, I began to press on the soles of the feet with a big file as I could find nothing else. I pressed on the top of the foot with the hands where the toes join the foot. I exerted this pressure over each foot for about three minutes at a time. The mother told me that the pressure on the feet gave her no pain whatsover.

"As she did not have any uterine pain, I was afraid there was no advancement. To my great surprise, when I examined her about 10 or 15 minutes later, I found the head within two inches of the outlet. I then waited about 15 minutes and found the head at the vulva.

"I then pressed again for about one or two minutes on each foot, the edge of the file being on the sole of the foot and my thumbs over the metatarsal-phalangeal joints as before. In this way I exerted pressure on the sole of the foot, and pressure on the dorsum (top) of the foot for about three minutes at a time, with my thumbs doing each foot separately for 1½ minutes. Within five or ten minutes the head was appearing, and I held it back to prevent tearing. It made steady progress, the head and shoulders coming out in a normal manner. Within three minutes the child—which "weighed in" at 9½ pounds—was crying lustily. The mother told me she did not experience any pain whatever, and could not believe the child was born. She laughed and said, 'This is not so bad!'

"Another point that is very remarkable is that after the child was born, the woman did not experience the fatigue that is generally felt, and the child was more active than usual. I account for this on the principle that pain inhibits (prevents) progress of the birth, and tires the child. But as the pain was inhibited, the progress was more steady, and thus fatigue to both mother and child was avoided.

Reflexology Used to Shorten Labor

A Massachusetts doctor supplements the above case with several others, equally revolutionary. To insure brevity and accuracy I quote the doctor's own words:

Case 1. Multipara (a woman who has had previous confinements), mother of four. Shortest previous labor eight hours. Had had a laceration of cervix (neck of womb) with her first child. Also one forceps delivery.

When labor commenced she was given two aluminum combs to hold and instructed to make strong pressure upon them with the view of inhibiting pains. The combs were to be used especially on the thumb and first and second finger. These combs were notched slightly and roughened on the ends so as to stimulate the side surfaces of the thumbs more effectively.

Was called at four a.m., arrived at 5:05, and the baby had just been born. The patient reported that she had been in bed for only 15 minutes. There had been one severe pain—that was when the head delivered.

There was no exhaustion following, as with previous labors, and she said laughingly, 'I believe I will be able to get up this afternoon, Doctor.'

The afterbirth delivery seemed to be stimulated, and the pains controlled by stroking the backs of the hands with the teeth of the combs. She became relaxed and drowsy from this stroking, and fell asleep and slept almost through the night, perfectly free from pain."

How Reflexology Caused an Unexpected Birth

A friend tells me the following story about her daughter's experience with reflexology:

A few weeks before my daughter's baby was due, I told her about the reflex method to painless childbirth as I had learned from you. I explained how to press the hands and fingers with a comb or solid object to relax the tension of the uterus when it was time for delivery, but I forgot to warn her not to use this method until she was sure that labor was starting and that her doctor was near.

They lived out in the country, and her husband was working about a half mile from the house.

This is what she told me. 'One afternoon as I lay on the couch to rest, I decided I would try the comb method you had told me about so that I would know how to do it when it was time for the baby. I got two ordinary combs, remembering that you had said they might break if one wasn't careful. I started pressing the teeth into my palms and then into my fingertips, just trying them out.

'I felt so quiet and relaxed after a few minutes I guess I just kept doing it. Then suddenly something broke in me and there was water all over everything—then I knew the baby was coming. I felt one little pain and there it was! I didn't know what to do. I wrapped it up in my husband's coat laying close by, and *walked* out to where he was working. He nearly fainted as he saw me all bloody. He rushed us to the hospital, and we were both fine. The next time I have a baby, I will use the combs and reflexology, but I will be sure I am not alone, and that someone is right there with me."

If you want to use the reflexology method to help you have a painless delivery, remember the experience of the above young mother and don't try it until you are sure that it is time for the baby to be born—and don't be alone.

HOW REFLEXOLOGY HELPS MOTHERS
BREAST-FEED THEIR BABIES

While we are talking about the advantage of painless childbirth, let's take one more look at the advantage of birth without medication and consider the future of the baby. We all know that breast-feeding is the most natural and healthful way of nourishing babies from birth to weaning time. We know that a substance in the human mother's milk protects infants against many infectious diseases.

A British doctor announced recently that "breast-fed babies are not nearly so susceptible to heart attacks when they grow to maturity. Breast-fed babies are susceptible to far less digestive trouble than bottle-fed ones."

Doctors Niles Newton and Michael Newton—a husband and wife team of psychologist and obstetrician, have devoted years to studying every aspect of breast-feeding as it affects mental and physical health of the infants and mothers. They are strong in their feelings about the necessity of breast-feeding for good psychological and physical health.

DELIVERY WITHOUT ANESTHESIA MAKES
IMMEDIATE BREAST-FEEDING POSSIBLE

These doctors claim that mothers have less trouble breast-feeding the baby immediately after birth with little or no anesthesia during delivery. It is not until the fifth or sixth day after birth that babies from heavily medicated mothers are able to nurse satisfactorily. Your baby needs complete nourishment a lot sooner then that to get a good start in life.

Bottle-fed Babies and Psychological Troubles in Later Life

And now we are told by these two experts on the subject that by depriving our babies of the experience of breast-feeding, we may be condemning them to a great deal of psychological trouble in later life, especially in the terms of sexual maturing and adjustment to the experience of having their own children.

There is no feeling in the world that can compare with the joy of holding your new-born baby close in your arms and feel his little mouth taking the nourishment from your body as nature intended.

Criminal Trends Caused by Non-Nursing Babies

Is it possible that much of today's violence and senseless crime may have its origin in depriving our children of the wholesome, natural, and instinctive act of nursing at mothers' breast?

If you are interested in this subject, you may write for a free manual to, "The Womanly Art of Breast-feeding." La Leche League, 3332 Rose St., Franklin Park, Illinois.

I give you this added information in the advantages of feeding the baby on the breast, hoping you will remember the experiences of the above-mentioned mothers when your next baby is born.

Have Painless Childbirth and Nurse Your Baby with Reflexology

Using Reflexology instead of medication when the baby is born can give you the experience of a painless and quick delivery plus the added chances of nursing your baby, thus promoting the health and happiness of you both, now and in the years ahead; and perhaps a greater chance for a better society tomorrow.

How I Relieved Pains of Pregnant Woman

A neighbor girl came over to my house one afternoon and asked if I would drive her to the doctor. Her husband was at work and we were 20 miles from town. I asked her what her trouble was. She said she was pregnant and had terrible pains in her side. She was only three months' pregnant, and I felt she had better see her doctor so I drove her the 20 miles to his office. He could not find anything wrong with her and told her it was just one of those things she would have to put up with.

I talked to her about reflexology and learned she had taken the treatments several times from a friend of mine near where she had lived. When we got home, I gave her a treatment. On her next visit to the doctor, she told him how the reflex treatments helped her and he said to continue them. All through her pregnancy the pain kept recurring at intervals, but the treatments stopped it for several days and sometimes for weeks. We never knew what had caused the pain which was located low down in her side. She had had a very bad time with her first baby, developing a heart problem and having to have several specialists.

I took her to the hospital when it was time for the baby. In view of the trouble she had with her last confinement, they had a heart specialist on standby.

She had the baby by Caesarean section with no complications whatsoever. We felt that the reflex treatments given during her pregnancy were responsible for the safe delivery of her baby, and for the fast, uncomplicated recovery and feeling of well-being in the following months.

39

Reflexology for Those Who Are Amputees

I have had so many ask what to do in case there is an arm or a leg missing. I will try to answer the question by telling you first to look at Charts #1 and #2 in the front part of this book.

You will see how the meridian lines run down through the full length of the body ending in the fingers and toes in Zone Chart #1. If a leg or an arm has been amputated, then the lines would follow through to the point where the limb or arm stops, but they would still go that far. Also look at Chart #2—the reflexes have to pass through the arms and legs to get to the hands and feet, but if the hand or foot is missing, then the reflex points would be in the end of the stump. They would be congested, to be sure, but they would still be there.

By experimenting a little, you will learn which method of massage is the most beneficial to you, either by holding a steady pressure on the tender reflex or using a gentle rotating massage. It might take a little probing to find them but it can be done and with very rewarding results.

If the area is very tender, then I would suggest you use the tips of your fingers to search for the tender spots. You will have no way of knowing which reflex button is giving you a signal of distress when you do feel a sore spot, but you can be sure it is calling for help, so massage the spot gently a few seconds; then continue your search for other distress signals. After awhile you will become quite adept at this and will learn which areas in your body the reflex buttons are stimulating.

After you have used the fingers to massage these reflexes for awhile, you may feel that you need to press a little deeper to get better results. In this case, some of the devices as described in another chapter may be helpful. You might find the Magic Reflex Massager would work well for you, or even the smooth teeth of the reflex comb might better serve your need; or even an eraser on a pencil might be helpful.

Anyway, keep trying, and I am sure you will be rewarded with the wonderful health results that others are getting.

40

How Reflexology Can Develop Your E.S.P. (Extrasensory Perception)

Anyone can use the simple technique of reflexology to develop his own natural powers of extrasensory perception.

Luciano Marchesi has devoted more than half his life to the study of parapsychology and has discovered through many years of experimenting that there are certain points on a person's body which, when stimulated, can release powerful mental forces.

By using the knowledge of stimulating these reflex points to develop extrasensory perception, Luciano Marchesi has unlocked the hidden mysteries of his mind and has unleashed strange powers. Marchesi claims there are more than 10,000 such sensitive spots on the body, many of them corresponding to those used by the Chinese in acupuncture. Thus they would also correspond with the reflex buttons we have been studying.

DIFFERENCE BETWEEN
ETHERIC AND PHYSICAL MASSAGE

In studying parapsychology, we learn that the human body is composed of two halves. The left side is the receiving side, and the right side is the transmitting side, according to Marchesi.

Remember that we do not use the same technique of sensitizing these E.S.P. points, which Marchesi calls "plaque," as we do when massaging the reflex buttons for health purposes. We are now dealing with the etheric channels and so we must use a light etheric touch with a metal object when stroking these psychic perception points.

USING REFLEX MASSAGE TO CONTROL YOUR DREAMS

Let us try a test which involves the gentle stimulation of the vertical cross "plaque" of clairvoyance which is found on the end of the third, or middle, finger of the left hand and located on the pad of the finger. To find the exact spot, draw a vertical line from the top of the finger to the first joint. Now draw a line across the middle of this line.

At night before you go to bed, take a pin and rub the head of the pin gently on this cross line of the middle finger, starting at the center where the vertical line runs and rub in one direction only. If you rub from the center of the finger toward the ring, or fourth, finger, you will dream of the future. If you stroke the pin head gently toward the index finger from the center line, you will dream of the past.

You might experiment with the metal comb or some other metal object in doing this exercise. You must relax while doing this, close your eyes, and concentrate. Do this for about half an hour before going to bed.

HOW TO DEVELOP VISUALIZATION OF OBJECTS

By using the receiving side of the body, you may also be able to develop your extrasensory powers to visualize certain unseen objects by viewing photos and also from holding or viewing certain objects.

To do this, you will draw a vertical line down the exact center of the palm of your left hand; now draw a horizontal line across the center of this line. Where they cross in the center of the palm is where your E.S.P. plaque is located. Now take a small metal object about a half-inch in diameter, preferably with a handle, or you might use a thimble. You can experiment with metal devices for this exercise. (Stirling Enterprises, Inc., in Cottage Grove, Oregon, might carry a device usable in E.S.P. experiments.)

Take the photograph or device you are going to use in this experiment and place it in front of you after holding it for a few moments.

Now, to invoke the magic of your extrasensory power, you will stimulate this ESP plaque in the center of the left hand by massaging it very lightly with the ESP device which you have chosen to use. When you are doing it correctly, you will feel a slight vibration, a prickling sensation, then a pain in the side.

Now you should be able to see or feel the deeper vibrations through the psychic perception which you are stimulating. At first you may get only faint impressions which will become stronger with practice.

Luciano Marchesi tells of one of his experiences using this exercise. A friend sent him a picture of a hilltop with a single bush on it. He stimulated the spot on his left hand and got the usual vibration of the prickling, then the slight pain in his side.

Then he saw something more in the photograph. The ground a few feet from the bush had once been lower. He could discern a small circular structure made of stone. A month later an excavation was begun, and the remains of a small circular Etruscan temple, 2500 years old, were found.

Here we are using reflex massage to help us develop psychic energy, thus enabling us to contact and use "Cosmic Awareness" and that Universal Sea of Wisdom which surrounds us all.

USING MENTAL FORCES TO HALT DECAY

Now let us look at the right side of the body which will be the transmitting side.

On your right arm, half-way between the wrist and the elbow, is a sensitive area about a half-inch in diameter, which, Marchesi calls a plaque. He states that this plaque enables one to project the mental force needed to halt decay.

The stimulation of several plaques by parapsychologists could be used to halt the progress of certain diseases and decay of the cellular system of psychological abnormalities.

He says he is not strong enough himself to halt decay in other than small things such as fish, tomatoes, and small animals, but feels that group techniques might possibly be used effectively for larger quantities of organic matter.

REFLEXOLOGY HELPS DEVELOP COSMIC POWERS
WITHIN US

Joseph Murphy, D.D., gives us many examples of using the extraordinary power of E.S.P. in his book, *Psychic Perception, The Magic of Extra-Sensory Power,*[1] such as how to see through walls, locate lost friends or relatives, receive wealth, visualize future events, etc.

But Luciano Marchesi is the first to give us a breakthrough on how to use a specialized form of reflexology to help develop the cosmic power within us.

Your body is an instrument or vehicle through which life-principle, or God, is expressed. Every person walking the earth is God, or life, in manifestation.

With a new vision, religion and science may both understand and use the mystic overtones of harmonizing the body and the psychic perception and you can learn to use the full forces of reflexing your E.S.P., so that you may achieve what you desire from life.

---

[1] West Nyack, N.Y.: Parker Publishing Company, Inc., 1971.

41

How to Rebuild New Cells with Reflexology

The famous Canadian doctor, Hans Selye ("The Stress of Life") said, "Life, the biological chain that holds our parts together, is only as strong as its weakest vital link."

You are as young or as old as your smallest vital links—the cells. The aging begins when your normal process of cell regeneration and rebuilding slows down. This slowdown is caused mainly by the accumulation of waste products in the tissues which interfere with the nourishment of the cells. Each living cell is a complete living entity with its own metabolism. It needs a constant supply of oxygen and sufficient nourishment.

HOW HEALTHY CELLS STOP PROCESS OF AGING

When our cells are deprived of fresh air, sufficient exercise and proper nourishment, they start to degenerate and break down. The normal process of cell replacement and rebuilding slows down and your body starts to grow old, in most cases before its time. Its resistance to disease will diminish and various ills will start to appear.

It is understandable that all of our glands, our bones, our skin, etc. are made up of these cells, so we must look first to the health of our cells.

Only about half of your cells are in the peak of development, vitality, and working condition. One fourth are usually in the process of development and growth, and the other three fourths are in the process of dying and replacement. The healthy vital life processes and perpetual youth are maintained when there is perfect balance in this process of cell breakdown and replacement. If the cells are dying at a faster rate than the new cells are built, the process of aging will begin to set in. It is of vital importance that the dying cells are decomposed and eliminated from the system as efficiently as possible. Quick and effective elimination of dead cells stimulates the building and growth of new cells.

Here is where reflexology comes in as the most effective way to restore your health and rejuvenate your body by the simple process of massaging the reflexes.

How to Eliminate Toxic Wastes with Reflexology

When you massage the reflexes you are sending a vital life force through the entire system, and reactivating the organs and the glands back to normal functioning. You are helping to clear out the sluggish metabolism and constipation, and the consequent inefficient elimination which causes retention and accumulation of toxic wastes in the tissues which interfere with the nourishment of the cells, causing disease and premature aging.

How to Replace New Cells for Old

Through this process of eliminating the toxic waste products by stimulating the eliminative glands with reflexology, their interference with the nourishment of the cells is effectively stopped, and the normal metabolic rate and cell oxygenation are restored, and you are on your way to replacing new cells for old! New cells mean new tissue and a new, rejuvenated body.

THE ELIMINATIVE GLANDS

You start this process of rebuilding healthy new cells by first increasing the eliminative and cleansing capacity of the eliminative organs—the lungs, liver, kidneys, and the skin. When these organs are reactivated by massage and pressure on the corresponding reflexes in the hands, masses of accumulated metabolic wastes and toxins are quickly expelled.

This is why we tell you to massage the reflexes for only a short time the first week or two, and not oftener than every other day the first week. When these organs start throwing off poisons, the concentration of toxins in the urine can be many times higher than normal. These eliminative organs begin to concentrate on the cleansing of old, accumulated wastes and toxins, such as uric acid, purines, etc., from the tissues.

How to Start Process of Rejuvenation

To start this process of rejuvenation you will give special attention to pressing and massaging the reflex to the liver. Massage the area of the pad under the little finger of the right hand, with the thumb of the left hand. Also don't neglect the web between the thumb and first finger. (See Figure 3 in the front of the book.)

Expel Toxins by Massaging Kidney and Lung Reflexes

Next we will go to the reflexes to the kidneys which are located near the center of both hands. If you are not sure, check Chart #2. See how the thumb is pressed into the kidney reflex in Figure 7 in the front of this book. Massage this a few seconds on each hand and then move up to the reflexes of the lungs which are located on the pads under the fingers. Check the chart for this if the position is not familiar to you. These also must be massaged on both hands.

Revitalizing Skin and Bones with Reflexology

Now we come to the skin, which is the largest part of our eliminative system since it covers our whole body structure.

You will note in Figure 41-1 how the hands are clasped. This is a natural stimulation to the whole nervous system.

By squeezing and releasing the fingers slightly several times you will be sending a flow of the vital life force through the whole body, including the skin and the bones.

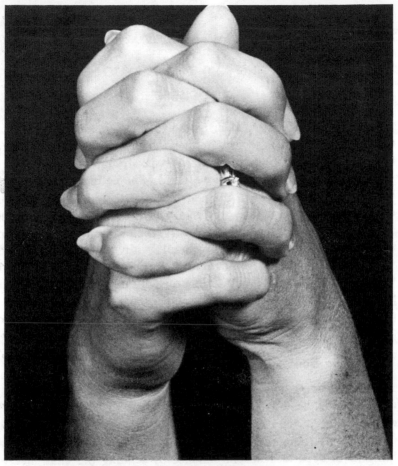

Figure 41-1. Position for relieving nervous tension by clasping the hands.

Stimulating All the Important
Elimination Reflexes

This is where the improved Magic Palm Massager is of great benefit, as it seems to stimulate all of these important elimination reflexes at the same time, and does a better job than just massaging one reflex at a time. When using the Magic Reflex Massager, be careful and don't over-massage the first time. This will not be easy to do—many people find it so stimulating they don't want to quit. So for the first week don't massage over two or three minutes at a time for each hand, no matter how good it feels.

227

BALANCING BODY CHEMISTRY TO HELP
CURE DISEASES

Alan H. Nittler, M.D., in his book, *New Breed of Doctor*, tells us, "It is 'tissue weakness' that opens the door to one new disease after another, and no drug can build tissue strength."

Disease is an abnormal condition of the cells and tissue caused by an abnormal balance of the body chemistry, and in this *abnormal condition* is the only place abnormal cells can live and grow. When there is a balance of the body chemistry, then normal cells are formed in which diseased cells cannot live and healthy tissue is able to grow.

If we regulate the glands into producing their normal secretion to balance the body chemistry, we are giving nature a chance to build perfect cells, thus making the environment unfavorable to the diseased cells.

Regulating Body Chemistry

In reflexology, we know that by stimulating certain reflexes, we can regulate the balance of the body chemistry by massaging the reflexes to all of the endocrine glands and organs. Whether the cause is from over-stimulation or under-stimulation, reflex massage will bring them back to a normal balance by sending the vital energy of life force into malfunctioning areas, thus regulating the chemistry of the body and giving nature a chance again to form normal cells in which the abnormal cells are no longer able to form.

I am not advising anyone to depend exclusively on any single remedy for a disease, but I do feel that what unnatural forces have disrupted, the healing forces of nature surely can put back into perfect working order.

In the book, *Edgar Cayce on Healing*, by Mary Ellen Carter and William A. McGary, M.D., there was some question of certain applications recommended by the great seer Edgar Cayce in many of his some 6,000 readings on healing. Edgar Cayce recommended Homeopathy (which is likened to Naturopathy, Osteopathy, and Chiropractic of today) as his choice of therapy. Remember that these recommendations came from a source which was not understood at that time and is just now being sought by those who are seriously seeking the answer to all diseases.

Edgar Cayce on the Aura

Here are some of the questions asked by the authors of *Edgar Cayce on Healing:* Is there an energy in the human body which we have not yet discovered? Is there an energy field around the body? Is this what has been called the aura?

Cayce described such a flow of energy in the form of a figure crossing at the area of the solar plexus. He also described the aura of the human being as ·being a type of force field visible only to those who can see it.

The practice of stimulating this energy life force to bring about therapeutic results has been used down through the ages, from the time of ancient Egypt.

MANY COUNTRIES USE METHODS RELATED
TO REFLEXOLOGY

Many countries use related methods of what we call reflexology to achieve healing of all types of diseases.

We know of the Chinese and their acupuncture, using the needle method; then there is the Ju-Jube of Africa, where they use quills dipped in herbs which are applied under and around the arms and armpits to tap these life currents.

Japanese have their method called *Shiatsu,* in which they use the fingers as in our western method of reflexology.

India also has her special method of using this ancient therapy to heal the body by stimulating the flow of the energy field, and many other countries have been using therapeutic methods related to reflexology down through the ages.

Do you know that in recent years Russian scientists have photographed energies spurting out of specific reflex areas? And that they have also photographed the aura; and that we are now able to do the same in this country?

These forces created by the human body are real and active.

They are, in fact, observable and recordable in all living things.

Reflex therapy not only acts on the muscular structures of the body but also performs therapeutic duty to the uncoordinated functional organism. By using reflex massage to all of the glands and organs, we balance the body so that its energies may be utilized in all its parts in restoration and regeneration of body tissues.

Cayce says that imbalance brings about certain glandular changes, particularly in the thyroid, which in turn disturbs the distribution of these energies or forces to their proper channels.

Cayce constantly talked of using the vibrations of several metals for healing, especially copper and iron to help activate the electrical energy forces. This is one of the reasons we recommend using the metal reflex combs for a better stimulation of the reflexes in the hands when practicing reflexology.

In her "Special Financial Forecast" for 1972-1973 Marguerite Carter, the great Unitology Forecaster tells us, "I believe with all my heart that we are on the threshold of the cure of diseases that are now taking so many lives, but the answer will not be 'new.' It is apt to be surprisingly simple and come about through a 'new way' of using something that has been at hand all along."

Many of us have sadly known of this forbidden secret for many years. But now, hopefully, under the pressure and the demand of the masses, the growing conscious and humanitarian feelings of many doctors, and a benevolent God, perhaps we are at last approaching the end to untold suffering and fear from so-called incurable diseases.

I will not tell you how to massage any certain reflex here, as I feel that you must concentrate on massaging the reflexes to all of the organs and glands, especially endocrine glands to achieve beneficial results. Study Chapter 12 on endocrine glands and your chart #3 and massage the reflexes as directed to help nature overcome illnesses of all kinds. It costs nothing and can do no harm, so at least try it.

I am constantly in search of new methods of natural healing, and when I find one that is better than the positive and simple methods of reflexology, I will bring this method to you.

You need no longer live in fear of so called incurable diseases: *nothing is incurable;* diseases are the result of malfunctioning of the cells and imperfection of the body tissues due to unnatural elements of living. Just turn to nature and give her a chance to put your body chemistry back into normal performance by rebuilding perfect cells and new healthy tissues for your whole body.

42

Relaxing Nervous Tension with Reflexology

Why do some people clench their teeth and double their hands into fists when they are upset or under emotional stress? When suffering great physical pain or when angry, they sometimes sink their teeth into their lips often hard enough to cause bleeding.

People perform these and many other natural acts of nature because they are instinctive and scientific, and because nature knows her business. We do them involuntarily and automatically because they relieve pain and nervous tension, and produce a form of analgesia, or pain-deadening effect.

Let us learn to use this release of tension by voluntarily using pressure on the reflexes as in Figures 4 and 18 in front of this book.

You will remember in Chart #2 how all of the fingers are marked "nerves," so you should massage the fingers to stimulate the nerves or use pressure on them to calm nervous tension.

If you are one of those people who live under nervous tension and anxiety, then you had better turn to nature's healing forces of reflexology and learn what it is like to live in peace and harmony even though there is strife and chaos all around you.

Quickest Way to Calm Nerves

The quickest, yet most inconspicuous method of calming the nerves, is to clasp your hands together as shown in Figure 41-1 and squeeze tightly. By looking at Chart #2, you can see how the act of pressing on all these nerve reflexes in the fingers at once must send a relaxing current into the whole system. While you have your hands clasped in this position, work the fingers back and forth; move all the fingers to above the second joint and press and roll them together again. If you will look at Figure 4 in the front of the book, you will see how the tips of the fingers are placed against each other. When doing this exercise, press as hard as you can and hold for a few minutes. By the time you finish this reflex exercise, you may wonder where all the nervous tension has vanished.

You may also use the metal massage comb to press and hold on the ends of the fingers and other places on the hands that seem to need pressure.

How Reflexology Helped Writer's Cramp

Dr. White tells of a case of neurosis—a writer's cramp—accompanying a neurasthenic condition. "This lady—unusually alert and intelligent—was a physical wreck. Sleepless, harassed by nerves in their most aggravated form, she was unable to hold a pen, or to write more than a few minutes at a time, until, on account of the pain and twitching of the arm, wrist, and fingers, she was forced to desist. She was also nearly deaf from a middle ear trouble.

"Several months' treatment, using the aluminum comb across the front and back of the hands and the finger tips, and daily employment of the tongue depressor (or probe) for four or five minutes, brought forth a complete change in the patient's condition

"It relaxed the terrible nervous tension—which was particularly marked along the course of the spine—enabling her to sleep at night, and awake thoroughly refreshed in the morning. The writer's cramp was completely cleared up. A number of other conditions were also corrected, and her hearing was improved by 50 percent.

"This lady has since resumed her occupation as a private secretary—a position she was forced by ill health to relinquish more than two years ago—and now writes for hours at a stretch without any return of the cramp in the hand and the arm."

How Reflexology Cures Neuralgia in Tongue

My mother had what the doctors called neuralgia in the nerve in her tongue. I have seen her tongue double back into her mouth in a spasm and she would scream with pain.

She went to many doctors who gave her opiates, not knowing of any other method of helping her. Finally, one doctor took her to a hospital in San Francisco and operated on her brain. He didn't help the nerve in her tongue, but cut a nerve to her throat which caused her to have severe choking spells. She had injections of Novocain in a nerve in her face which did help for a while.

Soon after I started to study reflexology she came to visit me, and at the suggestion of my teacher, I searched out a very tender place in her toe and massaged it. After the first few minutes of massage, the pain in her tongue stopped and never returned. Of course, I kept massaging this reflex as long as she was with me and I taught her how to continue massaging her toe after she went home. She has never had a recurrence of the terrible pain which caused her so much agony and trouble in the past.

How a Doctor Cured Tri-Facial Neuralgia

Doctor Roemer, gives this report of a tri-facial neuralgia patient being permanently relieved by his application of reflex pressure.

He tells of a man who came to him who had been suffering from tri-facial neuralgia for more than two years.

> The patient had been advised to have the nerve cut. He had been unable to speak or eat for five days because of the severe pain which radiated over the entire left side of the face extending to the lower jaw, the upper jaw and up into the left eye. The pain was of a sharp piercing nature." He goes on to tell us, "I applied rubber bands on the joint of the thumb and forefinger (which would be No. 2) of the left hand, and in less than ten minutes he was talking and laughing. Nothing was said to him about the pain or what the rubber bands were applied for. I told him to apply them every half hour if the pain continued, and as the pain grew less, to lengthen the interval of application. He continues to use the rubber bands once a day, 'so I won't get out of the habit and to make sure the pain does not return.' He is now enjoying life better than he has for years.

How Reflexology Stops Hand Tremors

Dr. White tells of a case of a young man suffering from hand tremors, insomnia, and nervous exhaustion. "He had his finger tips clamped daily for a week, then three times more, at intervals of three days. After the eighth treatment, he had no further trouble with the tremors, slept like a baby, and was apparently relieved of all nervous symptoms."

If you want to stop hand tremors, try putting the clamps on all the fingers for 15 minutes daily or more often, for one week, and see what happens. Clothespins may be used for this purpose, or rubber bands if you are able to watch them and remove them when the fingers begin to turn blue.

Clenching Teeth to Relax Nervous Tension

If you are extremely nervous, another method of producing a soothing degree of relaxation is to clench your teeth, if you have a good set, and also the hands for several minutes at a time, three or four times daily. You will find this method most helpful in overcoming nervous conditions.

Yawn and Stretch to Relax

Another one of nature's natural relaxing exercises is to yawn and stretch periodically. This exercise stimulates a healthy action of the sympathetic nerves in all the zones, and cannot fail to be of great benefit.

Using Reflexology to Cure Insomnia

If you are suffering from insomnia, try the following exercises after you are comfortably settled in bed. Interlock the fingers and clasp the hands, as shown in Figure 41-1, or press the finger tips firmly together, as shown in Figure 4 in the front of the book, holding this position for ten or 15 minutes, if you have not already fallen asleep by that time.

REFLEXOLOGY IMPORTANT FOR JET AGE

The most important thing in this jet age is to learn how to relax. Anything that will teach us to relax without drugs and sleeping pills will prove to be a boon to mankind. For this reason, I am certain that the principle of Reflexology will be a familiar and universally applied technique within the very near future.

Teacher Uses Reflexology
to Calm Nervous Tension

A teacher reports: "I want to tell you how Reflexology has helped me in working with children, both in the schoolroom and out in the playground.

"Children of today seem to be under a high tension. It takes a lot of patience and calm nerves to cope with them. I used to be in a continued state of nervous tension, but since discovering Reflexology, I can calmly handle any situation that arises. (Figures 9 and 15 in the front of the book).

"I 'keep my cool' as the children say, by massaging the nerve reflexes in my fingers and thumbs inconspicuously even while I am teaching.

"I only wish I could teach the art of Reflexology to the children. I am sure we would have healthier and happier children in the schools, and they would be better adjusted as adults in the future."

EXORCISM

A doctor sends me information on how to use reflexology to rid the body of possessions. It is a known fact by many that an entity from another dimension does take possession of a body, especially where the vibrations of the aura are lowered by alcohol or drugs.

How Doctor Uses Reflexology to Evict Possessions

Dr. Brandt told me that when a person is possessed by an entity, he has overactive adrenal glands. He says,

> The pancreas, the adrenal, the pituitary and the pineal are all doubly active, but by using reflexology to return these glands to normal, active functioning, it doesn't leave any room for the extra spirit in possession and he either starves or leaves.

This information should give those who are working with serious mental cases something to think about. The Bible tells of people being possessed, and in many cases today there is suspicion that certain individuals may be possessed; but no one will come out in the open and talk about it. I hope that the simple technique of using reflex massage on the endocrine glands will be tested by our doctors and psychiatrists in some of our sanitariums for the mentally ill.

For the success that I have had with these poor, confused people, I can only imagine the change that would take place in our institutions if the simple and harmless methods of reflex massage were used for a few weeks.

Forceful life pulsations are manifested in the regions of the mind and brain when the reflexes to these areas are massaged, also bringing help for many types of mental depression.

I brought my 86-year-old mother back to normal with the use of reflexology after she became senile from an operation. I know it works!

Radiation Burns Treated With Reflexology

"A doctor told me to write to you and send for the book, and that reflexology is akin to acupuncture and that all of this work was done by the ancient Egyptians.

"My husband had his legs burned by radiation and clots keep forming, and we have to keep working them out. I use the reflex treatments every night on him and they have helped very much. They have also relieved the pain of sciatica which he is very thankful for.

"I am having wonderful results with reflex massage and use it on all my friends that will let me. So grateful to you."

J.C., Texas

REFLEXOLOGY FOR CHILDREN

All children have a natural instinct to turn to nature for food, health and a way of life if they are given half a chance. This is why Reflexology is becoming so popular with the younger generation; even very young, pre-school children are able to give a treatment of reflex massage to their parents and members of the family. Many of these youngsters are quite fascinated by the response they get from a complaining relative.

Figure 23 in the front of the book shows how teenage girls are massaging reflexes in their friends' hands with a Reflex Rollo. Notice in Figure 11 how intense the small boy is in using the same massager on his own hand. He is using a child's natural instinct to find nature's method of maintaining good health.

How to Maintain Your Child's Health

To maintain the body in perfect health as the child is growing, the endocrine glands are of the most importance. If you feel that your child is not developing as he should, turn to the endocrine glands. If he seems to be growing too fast for his age, or not growing as fast as is normal, your doctor should be consulted. Then turn to massaging the reflexes to the endocrine glands, especially the pituitary gland. The reflexes to the pituitary will be found in the pad of the thumbs and also in the pads of the big toes. See the chapter on endocrine glands.

Many doctors are now encouraging the use of reflex massage since it is easy to do and can cause no harm when done as directed. Teach the child to massage these endocrine gland reflexes for himself. Nature will guide him to the right buttons and the correct pressure to use, once he has been taught how to use them. You will be amazed at his natural instinct to turn to reflexology in his search for a simpler and better way to health.

Children Use Reflexology to Help Others

Children can be taught to use the benefits of reflexology not only on themselves but also for others, to overcome such complaints as nervous tension, toothache, headache, eye strain, etc. It can be used to relieve pain in minutes when there is a need.

Reflexology can be used in cases of emergency, such as certain illnesses and accidents to alleviate pain until a doctor arrives.

Reflexology in Undeveloped Countries

Many of our younger people and also our older folks are going across the sea to bring light and comfort to those who are struggling in undeveloped countries. I hope they will take the knowledge and understanding of reflexology with them so that they may show how an act of nature can help them regain their health. I hope reflexology will be used and taught whenever possible in their travels.

Children Use Reflexology in Sports

Many children who are involved in the field of sports are learning to rub the nerve reflex centers in their fingers to relieve tension just before going into competition, even doing so inconspicuously during a game. See Figure 24 in front of book, showing a football player massaging his finger. He has learned that this quickly relaxes pent-up nerves, thus helping him enter the game calm and cool. He says it gives him a better chance of helping his team come out a winner.

Be a Winner with Reflexology

Reflexology will help you come out a winner every time if you will use it for any ailment or pain which might befall you. Don't leave this wonderful healing art for the younger generation to discover. Join them in their enthusiasm for nature's way to health through reflexology and you, too, will enjoy a fuller, happier way of life in perfect health for as long as you live.

Minister Encourages
Boy Scouts to Use Reflexology

Doctor Edwin F. Bowers relates that a minister, who taught his Boy Scouts "Zone Therapy" (Reflexology) methods with special reference to curing themselves of coughs and other common ailments, found it effective. He states further that the boys also found it valuable in their "First Aid to the Injured" work. One can readily understand that the analgesic effects of reflex pressure can be a factor in eliminating shock from pain whether in camp, at home, or a sudden onset of illness in the middle of the night when emergency help is not available.

To quote Dr. Bowers, "Zone Therapy opens up a tremendous field, so the more experiments we have, the sooner everyone will know just how tremendous and useful and marvelous it is."

43

How Rejuvenation Is Possible with Reflexology

Since time immemorial people have been looking for means of rejuvenation outside of themselves. They expected rejuvenation from witchcraft, the philosopher's stone, the fountain of youth, etc. The one place they forgot to search, where such possibilities have always been at hand, was within themselves.

RETURN TO YOUTH IS POSSIBLE

Who says we can't return to youth? Let me give you some facts of proof that it *is* possible to turn back the clock. I don't believe that man was meant to grow old and die so soon.

Prof. Hilton Hotema states, "Before the flood, men are said to have lived 500 and even 900 or more years. As a physiologist I can assert positively that there is no fact reached by science to contradict or render this as improbable. It is more difficult, on scientific grounds, to explain why man dies at all, than it is to believe in the duration of human life over a thousand years."

Ancient Masters Spoke of Rejuvenation

Some of the ancient masters often spoke of cases of rejuvenation, but their accounts have not been understood.

> "His flesh shall be fresh as a child's; he shall return to the days of his youth. And thy youth shall be renewed like the eagle's. These things worketh God oftentimes in man when man

knows how to live in harmony with the law." (Job 33; 25, 29: Psalms 103; 5)

Man's body is a materialization of the invisible gases of the air, consisting of electrolyzed and intelligized atoms. Man corresponds in color, number, and vibrations to the solar system at the moment of his birth. Man (you) becomes embodied in a prison of matter, and man's mind is inseparable from cosmic elements.

Your Youth Can Be Renewed Like the Eagle's

Your mind can, and does, control your body, and as soon as you believe there is hope for your renewed health and you start using God given natural ways to turn the clock back, then "shall your youth be renewed like the eagle's."

Dr. Alexis Carrel, who kept the cells of a chicken heart alive for 32 years said, "An organ is not made of (external) material, like a house. . . . It is born from a cell, and the body originated from one brick that would begin manufacturing other bricks from itself."

How a Man Out-Hikes His Son

Mr. D. tells of his dad using some kind of a stick to roll his feet on.

"I remember Dad sitting on the edge of his bed every night and rolling his feet on some kind of a stick. When I asked him what he did it for he just said the doctor told him to.

"Some years later when I came home from the Navy, my dad and I went on a hunting trip. He could out-climb me on every hill we came to. Up he would go like a mountain goat, while I puffed along behind him, with rests in between. He kept saying 'Come on, what is the matter with you, Frank?' He was a lot younger than I was physically. And I noticed he still rolled his feet on the stick every night.

"When I was introduced to the methods of Reflexology, I realized why my dad had been so energetic and healthy up into his late years."

87 Year Old Grandma Falls Downstairs

I gave a friend a book as a gift, and she said her 87-year-old grandmother borrowed it and never gave it back, "She thinks it is the most wonderful book she has ever read," L. tells me:

She uses it constantly on herself and everyone else including me, and it has helped all of us in many ways, yes, even the children. But let me tell you about Grandma falling down the stairs. She lives alone in her own house which has a basement where she does her washing. The other day Grandma came over and told me this story.

"I fell down the steps the other day into the basement." I was horrified, but I could tell Grandma was O.K. "What happened?" I asked. "Well, I opened the basement door and then turned to pick up some things I was going to take downstairs. I kind of got tangled up in some string on one of the boxes, and the next thing I knew, me and all those boxes and stuff were tumbling bumpety-bump down the steps.

" 'When I hit the bottom I just lay there a few minutes wondering if anything was broken. Then I started to wiggle my fingers and found out they were all right, then I wiggled my toes, then I started to rub my fingers and as soon as I could get myself untangled I also started massaging my feet. I didn't move from that floor for a good half hour until I had massaged every one of my reflexes good. Do you know I haven't even been sore from that fall? I wonder what I would have been like if I hadn't known about Reflexology?"

She credits everything to her reflex massage, and I will have to agree with her it is the greatest thing that has happened to this family.

Always keep in mind that reflex massage will absolutely relieve pain and, in most cases, remove the cause.

Nature has provided us with the necessities to sustain life and has generously given us this easy method of freeing ourselves from pain and ill health. Since we continually make use of all the other gifts of nature, we should gratefully accept her most precious gift, a healthy happy life through reflex massage.

How Aged Father Maintains Health

Although my father is quite old in years, because of his boundless energy people find it almost impossible to believe his true age. Since reading about reflexology, I think I know the answer.

Whenever he is sitting idly talking or watching television, he is constantly massaging his hands. He massages one hand completely with the thumb of the opposite hand pressed into the palm, while his fingers curl around and massage the back of the hand at the same time. He massages each hand in the same manner.

I realize now that he is instinctively using one of nature's most marvelous gifts, the reflex massage method of achieving and maintaining good health. I believe this inconspicuous method of keeping a vital life force of energy flowing through his body is the secret of excellent health and long life.

How Schoolteacher Calms Nerves

Another gentleman tells us of watching his schoolteacher place the tips of his fingers together and press them hard against each other several times a day while he was walking back and forth before his class and while sitting behind his desk. He was using a natural instinct to calm nerves and keep the forceful life pulsations manifested in the glandular regions of his body. He will probably remain in perfect health all of his life.

REJUVENATION BY MODERN PONCE DE LEON

An article in the Columbus, Ohio, *Dispatch* calls a San Francisco physician, Baron Andrew Von Salza (who is now retired in Santa Barbara, California), a contemporary "Ponce De Leon."

Dr. Von Salza, a very good friend of mine has helped me many times in my studies of natural methods to health. He is a specialist in rejuvenation, and studied the art of turning back the hands of time in Germany, Russia, and Italy. This modern Ponce de Leon was born in an ancient castle, built by his forefathers at the end of the nineteenth century in Thuringia, Germany. His parents emigrated to Russia where he studied at the University of St. Petersburg, then on to the University of Dorpat, Estonia, etc. The First World War interrupted his studies, but during the Second World War he worked in a biological research institute of experimental medicine which was created to study theories of rejuvenation. He worked with the highest

specialists on the subject and with pupils of such authorities as
Voronoff, Steinach, Alexis Carrel and others.

After escaping into the American Zone he developed a method
of his own rejuvenation system, called J2 therapy. In his book,
"Return To Youth," Dr. Von Salza tells us of many personalities,
including T.V. and movie stars who have returned to youth through
his natural method of reversing the process of aging.

Woman in Mid Sixties Has Healthy Baby

As proof that the hands of time can be turned back he gives this
account of an Austrian woman of 62, about 13 years post-menopausal.
On the tenth month of treatment she started menstruation normally.
On the thirteenth month of treatment she became pregnant and gave
birth to a healthy child who is now 12 years old. The woman is now
76 years old, but looks to be in her forties. He gives many accounts of
women and also men who actually *returned to youth.*

Seventy-two Year Old Man Regains Potency

He reports on Case #23, Male. High executive, 72 years of age,
underweight — 90 lbs at 5'5", no mental disturbances and perfect
heart. Arteritis obliterans along lower limbs, acute arthritis, arteriosclerosis with pronounced muscular atrophy. Parchment-like facial
skin. Unable to dress or walk, completely bedridden. Two years later:
weight 110, no sign of arteritis obliterans, no sign of muscular
atrophy, skin has healthy tan, very agile, got back his driver's license.
Potency returned with unusual vigor, something not experienced for
at least 20 years.

Famous Personage Dances After Treatment

Dr. Von Salza gives an account of his experience with
Reflexology. "Mrs. Carter's book on Reflexology is a welcome
addition to the field in preventing ailments as well as relieving
tensions and pains of a chronic nature.

"To test the worth of Reflexology I invited Mrs. Carter to
demonstrate her method of reflex massage on a famous person-

age, a patient of mine here in Hollywood, and was quite impressed with the result.

"My patient was in her late sixties, she could not move from one chair to another on the day of the treatment. The immediate improvement was quite astonishing and the aforementioned lady went to a night club in the evening and danced.

"I have enough faith in this method of healing to ask Mrs. Carter to open an office with my own. I believe that this is a simple and harmless method to health, and from my experience with Mrs. Carter I believe all that she says about Reflexology to be true."

Rejuvenation Therapy Used by Renaissance Spa

Now we learn that a spa has been opened in the Bahamas, by Dr. Ivan Popov, using the same rejuvenation therapy to reverse the process of aging which Dr. Von Salza has been using with such great success. Many of our most noted stars and people of society have undergone rejuvenation therapy at the Renaissance Spa in Nassau with fantastic results. They are overjoyed when these revitalizing treatments actually "Return Them to Youth."

Reversing the Process of Age

I don't claim that reflexology alone will do what these modern *Ponce de Leon's* are doing, but their experiences do give proof that reversing the process of age is possible, and by stimulating the cells with the vital magnetic life force from reflex massage you, too, have a chance to *Return to Youth.*

REFLEXOLOGY IS FOR EVERYONE

Reflexology is a boon to all mankind. You can use this rediscovered art of healing, not only to alleviate pain and many ailments on yourself, but also on others. Don't be afraid to massage any sore spots you may find on your hands or your feet; remember, *if it is sore, rub it out!* When there is pain any place in the body, follow the directions I have given in this book.

I am not a doctor, but through my lifetime of studying natural methods of healing, I give you the quickest and simplest method of helping yourself back to health through Reflexology. All you have to do is press the reflex buttons in your hands or your feet to start the healing forces of nature so that she may revive glandular activity.

Through the stimulation of these reflexes, you may be able to free yourself from pain and illness from this day on into your healthy happy future.

I give this book to you with compassion, knowing that it will reach out into the world and heal the anguished cry of deep despair and suffering for all who will once again turn back to nature for a way to live in perfect health the rest of your life.

INDEX

A

Acupuncture:
  ancient art of healing, 46
  can be dangerous, 46, 48
  premature use, 48
  reflexes agitated with needles, 82
  risk infection and injury, 50
  treats body as whole, 46
  versus reflexology, 46-50
Addicts, withdrawal, 146-147
Adrenals:
  alcoholism, 144-145
  arthritis, 163
  hypoglycemia, 140
  massaging reflexes in hand, 34, 60
  one atop each kidney, 154
  possession, 236
  thumb in center of hand, 92
Airola, Paavo O., 161
Alcoholism:
  adrenal reflexes, 145
  carbohydrates not properly
      metabolized, 144
  compared with diabetes, 144
  deficiency in adrenal cortical
      hormones, 145
  energizing endocrine system, 145
  glandular disorder, 144
  low blood sugar, 144
  malfunctioning adrenal
      glands, 144-145
  massaging, 145-146
  misunderstood disease, 146
  pancreas and liver reflexes, 145
  pituitary gland, 145
  pituitary reflexes, 145
  too much insulin, 144
Alimentary canal:
  bile, 135
  bile duct, 135
  caecum, 135
  cutting up and grinding food, 133
  duodenum, 135
  gall bladder, 135
  glycogen, 135

Alimentary canal: (cont.)
  gullet, 133
  how gastric juices are
      produced, 133, 135
  how liver functions, 135
  large intestine, 135
  moistened, softened food, 133
  pancreas produces insulin, 135
  peritoneum, 135
  rectum and anus, 135
  reproductive organs, 204, 205
  salivary glands, 133
  small intestine, 135
  solid fats converted, 135
  starch converted into sugar, 135
  teeth, 133
  tongue, 133
  water, 135
  way body uses sugar, 135
Allergies, 149
Amputees, 218-219
Anemia, 95-96
Anesthesia, 82, 83, 123
Animals:
  asthmatic dog, 88-89
  hip operation on horse, 87
Anus, 135
Appendicitis, 148-149
Appendix:
  location of reflex, 28-30
  massaging reflexes, 60
Arm, aching, 76
Arteriosclerosis, cerebral, 141
Arthritis:
  affects entire body, 161
  alleviate pains and aches, 160
  backache, 112
  biochemical structure of body
      tissues, 161
  "biochemical suffocation," 161
  degenerative disease, 160
  endocrine glands, 161
  foot, 165
  glandular disorders, 161
  halt further damage, 160
  hand massager, 162

Ear: (cont.)
  reflex clamp, 83
Edgar Cayce on Healing, 228-229-230
Eliminate glands, 225-226
Emphysema, 174-176
Endocrine glands:
  adrenals, 92
  alcoholism, 144-146
  arthritis, 161
  chart, 28-30
  children, 90, 93
  ductless, 90
  giant or dwarf, 90
  gonads (sex glands), 92-93
  hormones secreted into
    bloodstream, 90
  hypoglycemia, 139
  interrelated, 90
  pancreas, 92, 136-137
  parathyroids, 92
  pineal, 91
  pituitary gland, 90
  supplement and depend upon
    each other, 90
  thymus, 91
  thyroid, 91
  vital life forces, 93-94
  well-being of individual, 90
Epilepsy, 138
Etheric massage, 220-221
Exorcism, 236-237
Extrasensory perception:
  comb, 221
  "cosmic awareness," 222
  decay of cellular system, 222
  develop cosmic powers, 223
  diseases, 222
  dreams, 221
  etheric and physical
    massage, 220-221
  left side receives, 220-221
  Marchesi, Luciano, 220-223
  middle finger, 221
  palm, 221
  "plaque," 221
  psychological abnormalities, 222
  right side transmits, 220-222
  visualization of objects,
    221-222
Extremities, lower, 79
Eyes:
  blocked circulation, 180
  cataracts, 183-184
  diabetes, 180
  fatigued nerves, 180
  faulty kidneys, 180
  itching, 182

Eyes: (cont.)
  location of reflexes, 27, 30,
    180-181
  massaging eye reflexes, 181-182
  massaging reflexes in hand, 58
  optic nerves, 182
  reflex clamp, 84, 85
  right, 37, 40
  stimulate reflexes around, 181
  strain, 181
  tension, 34
  watery, 183
  weakness, 156, 180

F

Fallopian tubes, 202
Fats, solid, 135
Female disorders, 112
Fingernails, 196
Fingers:
  eye and ear reflexes, 30
  massaging fronts and backs, 56
  No. 2 and No. 3, 56-57
  No. 4 and No. 5, 57
  reflexes stimulate head
    area, 55-57
Fitzgerald, 49 62, 63, 167
Foot, arthritis, 165
"Forever Young, Forever Healthy," 93
Fredericks, Carlton, 138, 141

G

Gall bladder, 60, 125, 135
Gastric juices, 127, 133, 135
Giant, 90
Glucose tolerance test, 141
Glycogen, 135
Gonads, 92-93, 140, 163
Goodman, Herman, 138, 141
Gullet, 127, 133
Gyland, Stephen, 141

H

Hair:
  baldness, 197-198
  barometer of health, 196-197
  falling, 196-198
  gray, 197
  growing, 196-198
  modified skin structure, 196
  nails, 196
  protein, 196
  regrowth, 38
Hand Massager, 124, 140, 162

Pancreas: (cont.)
small islands which secret insulin, 136
stimulate reflexes to other endocrine glands, 137
Parathyroids:
arthritis, 162
compression massage on fingers, 103
congestion, 103
foot massage simplest, 102
functions, 92
how hard you press, 103
location, 102
massager, 102-103
pencil with an eraser, 103
poise, tranquility, well-being, 103
size, 102, 103
two on each side of thyroid, 102
Pepsin, 126
Peptic ulcer, 138
Peritoneum, 135
Physical massage, 220-221
Pinched nerve, 98
Pituitary gland, 28, 90, 140, 145, 162, 201, 203
"Plaque," 221
Possessions, 236-237
Pregnancy, 157, 216
Prolapsed rectum, 153
Prostate gland, 36, 209
Protein, hair, 796
Psychological abnormalities, 222
Psychosis, 138

R

Radiation burns, 237
Rays, metal, 69
Receiving, 220, 221
Rectum, 135, 153
Reflex clamp:
aching tooth, 178
anesthesia, 82, 83
arthritis, 162
back troubles, 83
bladder, 158
childbirth, 83
deafness, 83
drug withdrawal, 146-147
ears, 186
easy to use, 85
eyes, 84, 85, 181
heart, 117
kidneys, 157
liver, 32
reproductive organs, 202, 203

Reflex clamp: (cont.)
ring finger of left hand, 83, 84
safe for any age, 85
stomach, 128
stroke, 120
voice, 192
Reflex Hand Massager, 181
Reflexology:
analgesic in minor operations, 49
ancient art of healing, 46
animals, 88-89
basic simplicity, 50
can be used by anyone, 47
conditions requiring other therapy, 50
curing anesthesia, 82
head, neck and shoulder pains, 104
health benefits, 49-50
mind can influence body, 86
network of channels, 50
not subject to man-made restrictions, 48-49
proof, 86-89
scientific, 47
simple, harmless method, 47
stimulates *Golden Cord of Life,* 50
tongue, 66-67
versus acupuncture, 46-50
what it is, 47
Rejuvenation, 240-246
Reproductive organs:
adrenals, 204, 205
arthritis, 163-165
cancer, 199
clamps, 202, 203
comb technique, 207
cysts on cervix, 199, 200
fallopian tubes, 202
first finger, 202
hormones, 201
hot flashes, 208
importance of sex glands, 201
lower lumbar area, 201, 202
"Lydia Pinkham," 200
Magic Massager, 202, 205
miscarriage, 208
pain quited, 203-205
painful menstruation, 207
pituitary gland, 201, 203
position of sex glands and organs, 201
profuse menstruation, 207
prostate, penis, uterus, 201-203
renewed interest in sex, 80
rubber bands, 203